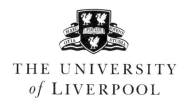

THE UNIVERSITY
of LIVERPOOL

Carers' Guide to Physical Interventions and the Law

Information and advice for parents, carers and care workers supporting children, young people and adults with learning disabilities

Professor Christina M Lyon and Alexandra Pimor

British Library Cataloguing in Publication Data

A CIP record for this book is available from the Public Library

ISBN 1 904082 81 5

© 2005 Professor Christina M Lyon and Alexandra Pimor

BILD Publications is the imprint of:
British Institute of Learning Disabilities
Campion House
Green Street
Kidderminster
Worcestershire DY10 1JL

Telephone: 01562 723010
Fax: 01562 723029
E-mail: enquiries@bild.org.uk

Website: www.bild.org.uk

This Carers' Guide is a companion to the full report *Physical Interventions and the Law: legal issues arising from the use of physical interventions in supporting children, young people and adults with learning disabilities and severe challenging behaviour* by Professor Christina M Lyon and Alexandra Pimor, also published by BILD. For a publications catalogue with details of all BILD books and journals telephone 01562 723010, e-mail enquiries@bild.org.uk or visit the BILD website www.bild.org.uk

DISCLAIMER

COPYRIGHT PROTECTION

BILD Publications are distributed by:
BookSource
32 Finlas Street
Cowlairs Estate
Glasgow G22 5DU

Telephone: 08702 402 182
Fax: 0141 557 0189

Acknowledgements

Professor Lyon and Alexandra Pimor would like to acknowledge here the contributions made by a wide range of individuals and organisations. It should be noted, however, that a number of other individuals who made specific contributions to particular parts of the text are acknowledged at that part of the text and are not referred to again here for reasons of space, but we would like to take this opportunity to thank them all for their help.

Among those groups and individuals whom we would particularly like to thank are: various officials at the Department of Health and the Department for Education and Skills who gave of their time and advice so freely; John Harris and all the members of staff at BILD (British Institute of Learning Disabilities); George Matthews and all the members of staff at Team-Teach; David Leadbetter and all the staff at CALM Training; all the members of staff at Studio 3; Patrick Crawley, Trevor Dickens and Margaret Townley, Training Officers with Nottingham City Social Services, for providing Professor Lyon with the opportunity to meet the enormously dedicated work force of Nottingham City Social Services; Professor David Allen, Consultant Clinical Psychologist and Honorary Professor at the Welsh Centre for Learning Disabilities; and Marion Cornick of the Loddon School, Hampshire; for all of their very helpful and informative comments on the drafts; various subscribers to the Mental Health Policy Forum run by Neil Morris of the Learning Disabilities Foundation; various members of VOICE UK; Anne Morris of the University of Liverpool Law School for reading and commenting upon the Employer's Liability sections, although any errors of law remaining are entirely our responsibility; and finally Vanessa Muir of the Devon Partnership National Health Service Trust.

Finally, we would both like to acknowledge the huge debt of gratitude we owe to Clare Dickinson, who has so ably produced and made sense of our manuscript and produced the final copy of the *Physical Interventions and the Law* report and this Carers' Guide.

Contents

Preface

Professor Chris Jones

The Impact of the 1994 Report entitled *Legal issues arising from the care and control of children with learning disabilities who also present with severe challenging behaviour* and the Parents and Carers Guide of the same name.

In 1992 the Mental Health Foundation commissioned Professor Christina Lyon to consider the legal issues arising from the care, control and safety of children with learning disabilities who also presented severe challenging behaviour. The purpose of that work was to consider legal issues arising from the provision of services to such children as well as from the use of physical interventions in providing for the care of such children. At the time, she was serving on the Foundation's Committee which in 1997 produced its own Report on the poor state of services for such children in England and Wales entitled *Don't forget us* in which Professor Lyon also wrote the chapter on legal issues. It emerged during that Committee's investigations that there were a huge number of myths concerning the legitimacy of the use of physical interventions as a result of the implementation, in October 1991, in England and Wales of the Children Act 1989.

For this reason, as Alan Jefferson noted in his Foreword to Professor Lyon's main 1994 Report, the Committee in 1992 commissioned Professor Lyon to produce a report enabling those providing such care to be clearer about the legal implications of Government Guidance as well as of then current and emerging practices. A full *Research, Policy and Guidance Report* and a *Parents and Carers Guide*, were published in 1994 by the Mental Health Foundation. The influence and impact of the 1994 documents were very considerable. The Mental Health Foundation constantly had to order reprints of the report even as late as 1999. Even more interesting was the warmth of the welcome extended to the two documents by Government bodies such as the Department of Health and the Department for Education and Skills. Departmental representatives on the Mental Health Foundation Committee had been intensely sceptical that such guidance could be produced since, in their experience, government lawyers like local authority lawyers had been very reluctant to give advice on such issues.

The impact of the 1994 documents can be seen today: in numerous documents produced by BILD, in the work of training organisations and in the Department of Health and Department of Education and Skills' own 2002 *Guidance on the Use of Restrictive Physical Interventions* which is the subject of detailed examination in Chapter 4.2 of the main Report. Thus, several paragraphs and examples given throughout the current DfES/DoH Guidance are derived from the 1994 documents, for example in the underlying principles at page 4, and at paragraphs 3.3, 3.5, 4.1, 6.1, 8.1 and 8.2, 9.1 9.3, 10 generally, 11, 12 and 13. The 'TINA' approach, that of resorting to physical interventions only when 'there is no alternative' was used first by Professor Lyon as it was the short name by which she had been known since childhood.

She first used it in training in 1981 to suggest the 'TINA' approach now used by a variety of trainers across the country. In addition, the recently proposed Mental Incapacity Bill for England utilises many of the approaches first put forward by Professor Lyon in the 1994 documents. Originally, Professor Lyon entered discussions with David Ellis at the DoH to ensure that when the new Guidance emerged, this Carers' Guide as well as the main Report, which is intended to aid in its interpretation, would be immediately available. Initially, the Department expressed an interest in funding the work but unfortunately, due to a shortage of resources, central government funds were not available. John Harris at BILD then gathered together a consortium of funding bodies to finance the production of the new *Physical Interventions and the Law* report and *Carers' Guide to Physical Interventions and the Law*.

The 2004 report and guide for carers

This new Guide deals with the law in England and Wales and covers not only children but also young people and adults. The main Report covers the law in Scotland as well but it has not been possible to produce a carers' guide to cover all the UK jurisdictions as this would have been far too long. With changes in the law occurring so rapidly, including the very recent implementation (on 15 January 2005) of Section 58 of the Children Act 2004, restricting the rights of parents to raise the defence of reasonable chastisement when punishing their children, it takes a lot of effort to ensure that Guidance like this is as up to date as it possibly can be. Working with Christina as I still am, and formerly with Alex, in the Centre has meant that I have had a opportunity to observe closely the painstaking efforts in which they engaged to ensure that this new Guide as well as the main Report will be of the greatest value possible to those who support children, young people and adults with learning disabilities and challenging behaviour. I commend this work to all those who work with and support such children, young people and adults.

Professor Chris Jones

Professor of Sociology, Social Policy and Social Work, Department of Sociology, Social Policy and Social Work, Co-Director of the Centre for the Study of the Child, the Family and the Law, University of Liverpool

Chapter 1

Employer's liability

Introduction

This chapter outlines the responsibilities and duties an employer owes to his employees and third parties. Employer's liability is an important area of the law which people who work with individuals with learning disabilities and severe challenging behaviour should have a basic understanding of in order to be familiar with the duties and responsibilities within which they work.

Criminal vicarious liability

The general rule is that a person is responsible for his own actions and not for the actions of another, as supported by case law dating back to 1730, which provides that: 'each answer for their own acts and stand or fall by their own behaviour'.

However, there are occasions where an employer can be liable for the acts of his employee. When an employer gives his employee specific instructions to carry out a certain task and the employee does as directed, but doing so actually amounts to committing an unlawful act, the employer would be held liable for the employee's action. Therefore, for an employer to be charged as a consequence of the act of his employee, there must be an instruction by the employer to the employee to carry out the illegal act.

Civil liabilities

Civil vicarious liability   An employer can be found liable for the wrongful civil acts of his employees when the acts were committed in the course of their employment. There are three components to the principle of vicarious liability: the wrongful act must be a tort, committed by an employee, in the course of his employment.

Employer's liability   An employer owes a duty of care towards his employees, which includes taking the necessary steps to avoid the latter incurring injuries and/or being subjected to violence in the workplace; and is under a common law duty to provide his employees with a) competent work colleagues; b) a safe place of work; c) proper plant and equipment; and d) a safe system of work.

Statutory duties   A statutory duty is an explicit obligation or prohibition to perform a duty in a specified manner enacted by Parliament. The Act in question also often provides guidance on adequate remedies available for a breach of such duty; alternatively, there may be other means of enforcement, such as common law remedies.

Health and Safety

The **Health and Safety at Work Act 1974** is an important piece of legislation, which applies to the whole of the United Kingdom and is the basic legal source on health and safety matters in any work activity. The main obligation imposed by this piece of legislation is that efforts must be made 'so far as is reasonably practicable' to ensure that every measure is taken to avoid employees and third parties coming to harm due to work-related risks. The Act is supported by two sets of regulations, in particular, which are relevant to the present guide: the **Manual Handling Operations Regulations 1992** and the **Management of Health and Safety at Work Regulations 1999**.

The Act and subsequent regulations all require that employers carry out risk assessments to establish what the potential risks are associated with any proposed action and how they can be tackled. The evaluation of work-related risks must then be supported by, and laid out in, policies and made available to all relevant parties, including employees, relevant third parties and possibly members of the public.

Responsibility to provide P.I. training

Paragraph 13.1 of the recent DoH/DfES *Guidance on the Use of Physical Interventions*[1] provides that:

> *'staff who are expected to employ restrictive physical interventions will require additional, more specialised training. The nature and extent of the training will depend upon the characteristics of the people who may require a physical intervention, the behaviours they present and the responsibilities of individual members of staff.'*

The *Guidance on the Use of Physical Interventions* also stresses the point that any physical techniques used must be selected according to the characteristics and the needs of each individual who presents the challenging behaviour. Once trained, a support worker must only use the techniques which he was taught in the manner in which he was taught and cannot modify them (paragraph 13.2).

Risk assessment

Risk assessment plays a vital part in any discussion on the possibility of introducing the use of physical intervention as part of an individual's care plan in response to a challenging behaviour, and must also be incorporated in a policy statement on physical restraint so as to give staff guidelines on recognising and preventing risks in certain given situations.

The Health and Safety Executive has provided a leaflet which spells out the five steps which employers are advised to follow when conducting a risk assessment:[2] 1) look for hazards; 2) decide who might be harmed and how; 3) evaluate the risks and decide whether the existing precautions are adequate or whether more should be done; 4) record your findings; and finally 5) review your assessment and revise it if necessary.[3]

Although the guidelines are not compulsory, they are a good indication of what would constitute good practice, and thus of what would be accepted as such in a court of law.

Violence at work

The five steps to risk assessment also apply in situations where staff are at risk of incurring injury due to voluntary or involuntary aggressive behaviours aimed at their physical integrity. The relevant legislation is the Health and Safety at Work Act 1974; the Management of Health and Safety at Work Regulations 1999; the Reporting of Injuries, Diseases and Dangerous Occurrences Regulations 1995; the Safety Representatives and Safety Committees Regulations 1977; the Health and Safety (Consultation with Employees) Regulations 1996; and The Manual Handling Operations Regulations 1992, as well as relevant European Community Directives.

The Department of Health's National Task Force on Violence Against Social Care Staff[4] provides guidelines to employers on their responsibility as regards violence at work; and a checklist to guide employees both on their own responsibilities and their employer's duties and responsibilities. In brief:

Employees must:	Employers have a duty to provide employees with:
Familiarise themselves with their organisation's various procedures, and with what triggers 'risk' situations	A policy statement and risk assessments
Be prepared to gather, share and discuss information on 'risk' situations/service users; and to go on appropriate training programmes	Procedures on what to do in a risk situation and procedures to check and review safety precautions Appropriate training, safe working environment
Use risk assessment and re-assess the risks	Support for employees' concerns over abuse and violence, and after a violent incident
Plan what employees and others will do, including the participation of managers, service users and carers	
Be prepared for unexpected, uncommon and otherwise rare violent incidents	

Chapter 2

Criminal law offences

Introduction

This chapter examines potential criminal liabilities which may face parents, carers and other individuals working with people with learning disabilities and challenging behaviour when they find themselves in situations where they need to use physical interventions on the people they care for.

Offences against the person

False imprisonment   False imprisonment consists of the unlawful and intentional or reckless restraint of a victim's freedom of movement from a particular place. Merely preventing an individual from taking a certain direction, however, when he can take another in order to reach his chosen destination will not amount to false imprisonment.

Common assault   Assault is the act of causing a person to fear for their physical safety and to apprehend the application of immediate unlawful violence upon them. If one is working with people with learning disabilities, one must be aware of the possibility that they may have fears about particular courses of action which others without learning disabilities might not have.

An assault does not require actual physical contact (as opposed to battery); however, the person committing the assault must either intend to apply physical touching, or be reckless as to whether they cause the victim to fear such an outcome. A mere omission to act will not necessarily amount to an assault – unless it is part of a continuing act. Finally, the use of words can be sufficient to constitute an assault.

Battery   The offence of battery will always include the offence of assault. However, the reverse is not always true, as an assault does not necessarily include an offence of battery.

Whereas the offence of assault can be committed by the threat of violence, battery is concerned with the *actual application* of force upon a person, whether it is intended or reckless. Any unlawful physical contact, including the slightest touching, can amount to battery. Consequently there is no need to prove that harm or pain has been caused.

Battery can occur even when the touching is not directly applied onto the physical body. As such, a support worker can commit a battery just by touching or grabbing the clothes of the person they support and whether the latter is aware of the touching or not is irrelevant.

Another indirect application of force that can constitute a battery is when the act of a support worker that is directed at one individual actually affects another, causing the latter to be subjected to unlawful personal violence upon them.

Assault occasioning actual bodily harm   This offence is set out in Section 47 Offences Against the Person Act 1861. Actual bodily harm is described as any hurt or injury that has intentionally been inflicted on an individual to affect their physical health and well-being. Actual bodily harm need not cause an injury that has permanent or serious consequences, nor is it necessary that actual bodily harm be proved by physical marks such as bruises. However, the injury must be significant, that is, it must cause sufficient pain or discomfort to the victim. Psychological harm can qualify as actual bodily harm (eg shock) provided it is not mere strong emotions (eg fear, distress, panic).

Malicious wounding/inflicting grievous bodily harm   Malicious wounding or inflicting grievous bodily harm, contrary to Section 20 Offences Against the Person Act 1861, does not necessarily require violence. Therefore, assault and battery need not be present for an offence of maliciously wounding or inflicting grievous bodily harm to be actionable. Furthermore, this means that psychiatric injury, which does not always include physical violence, comes within the ambit of Section 20 Offences Against the Person Act 1861. Although grievous bodily harm is to be understood as 'really serious harm' it does not mean that the harm has to be life threatening and 'wounds' implies that there is a discontinuity in the whole of the skin. In other words, a cut will amount to wounding.

Intention or subjective recklessness in maliciously wounding or inflicting grievous bodily harm must be proven, 'maliciously' implying that the offender was at least aware of the potential risk and consequences of applying unlawful force.

Wounding/causing grievous bodily harm with intent contrary to Section 18 Offences Against the Person Act 1861   Since the meaning of 'cause' is broader than that of 'inflict', it is sufficient for the act of violence to be proven substantial in causing the wound. Here, 'wound' and grievous bodily harm have the same meaning as in Section 20 Offences Against the Person Act 1861. Section 18 is distinguished from Section 20 as Section 18 requires proof that the unlawful act is done with the specific intention of causing really serious harm.

Homicide

Murder   Although there is no statutory definition available, it is found in common law that a murder is an act by which a person takes the life/causes the death of another – a human being – with malice aforethought. Malice, here, means that there is an intention to kill or at least an intention to cause grievous bodily harm.

Voluntary manslaughter   Voluntary manslaughter is an act that can be described as murder; however, the court will look at mitigating circumstances that will serve as partial defence and thus reduce the offence from murder to manslaughter and the resulting life sentence to a certain amount of years of imprisonment.

Voluntary manslaughter, like murder, is the intentional unlawful killing of a human being. However, the crime is reduced from murder to manslaughter on grounds of provocation, diminished responsibility or death being caused in pursuance of a suicide pact.

Involuntary manslaughter Involuntary manslaughter is also akin to murder, however the difference is that there is no intention to deprive the victim of their life. The homicide is due to an unlawful act but the offender did not intend to kill nor impose grievous bodily harm on the victim; therefore, this offence covers 'accidental murders'.

Chapter 3

Civil law torts

Introduction

This chapter is concerned with the potential liabilities parents, carers and other individuals working with people with learning disabilities and severe challenging behaviour may face under the civil law of torts where physical interventions have been employed to deal with challenging situations.

Assault

An assault is an act which makes the victim fear the application of immediate personal violence. The victim need not be touched or come to actual physical harm, nor is it important to determine what the wrongdoer actually intends. It is enough that the victim is under the impression that they will be subjected to imminent violence.

Battery

The tort of battery occurs when a person intentionally and directly applies unlawful physical contact against another individual. Injury need not be a consequence of this act; nor is force a requirement. In medicine, for instance, a treatment which is imposed on a person without their consent may amount to a battery. The application of physical touch must be intentional. In the absence of intention, the act becomes a matter of negligence.

False imprisonment

The tort of false imprisonment is committed when a person intentionally and directly restrains another's freedom of movement. This includes unlawful arrest and unlawful prevention of a person leaving a particular place (eg room, open field). The tort can still occur whether the claimant is unconscious or unaware that they are being restrained at the time. The restraint must be a direct consequence of a positive act. Thus, it will not be false imprisonment if it is the result of a careless action. Force is not required for this tort as words alone can give rise to a false imprisonment.

Negligence

Negligence has been defined as a tort consisting of a legal duty to take care on the part of the defendant and a failure to do so, thus resulting in a breach of duty, which causes the plaintiff to suffer harm. The tort of negligence is comprised of four main elements, which are a) that the defendant owes a legal duty of care to the plaintiff; b) the defendant has breached this duty by falling below the required standard of care demanded of him; c) the plaintiff has suffered harm or damage as a result of the breach of duty; and d) the damage or harm suffered by the plaintiff was not too remote (ie could have been anticipated.)

Chapter 4

Human rights law breaches

Introduction

The protection of an individual's human rights has become a fundamental obligation for the UK domestic courts since the implementation of the Human Rights Act 1998. This chapter aims to give an overview of the provisions which are particularly relevant to people with learning disabilities and severe challenging behaviour, and with which parents and carers should familiarise themselves.

Impact of the Human Rights Act 1998 particularly relevant to physical interventions

Article 2 – Right to Life   This Article aims, on the one hand, to safeguard individuals against arbitrary deprivation of life by public authorities, and on the other hand, to impose upon the State a responsibility to protect individuals against unlawful killings. However, the European Court of Justice has found that Article 2 does not guarantee individuals a right to die or to choose to die (see *Pretty v UK* 2002[5]).

Article 3 – Prohibition of Torture and Inhuman or Degrading Treatment   The State has a duty to protect people against the threat and/or inflicting of torture and inhuman or degrading treatment or punishment. In *A v UK* 1999,[6] the United Kingdom was found to have failed to protect a 9-year-old boy from being beaten by his father. This case established a positive duty on the part of the UK Government to enact laws and to take appropriate steps to help prevent an individual from suffering from degrading treatments or punishments.

Torture

In Article 1(1) of the Convention against Torture and Other Cruel, Inhuman or Degrading Treatment or Punishment, which was adopted by the General Assembly of the United Nations in December 1984, 'torture' is defined as:

> *'Any act by which severe pain or suffering, whether physical or mental, is intentionally inflicted on a person for such purposes as obtaining from him or a third person information or a confession, punishing him for an act he or a third person has committed or is suspected of having committed, or intimidating him or coercing him or a third person, or for any reason based on discrimination of any kind, when such pain or suffering is inflicted by or at the instigation of or with the consent or acquiescence of a public official or*

other person acting in an official capacity. It does not include pain or suffering arising from, inherent in or incidental to lawful sanctions.'

Inhuman or Degrading Treatment

An inhuman treatment is a premeditated action that is applied to an individual for a lengthy and continuous period of time and that causes the person to suffer either actual bodily injury, physical and/or mental harm. Moreover, a degrading treatment is an act which inspires in the victim such feelings as fear, anguish and inferiority, which are capable of reducing the latter to a state of humiliation and debasement. Finally, the suffering or humiliation endured by the victim must be so serious that it goes beyond the suffering and/or humiliation to be expected from 'a legitimate form of legitimate treatment or punishment'.

Inhuman or Degrading Punishment

A degrading punishment, which occurs when a person is treated as an object by the authorities, is considered as an 'assault on the person's dignity and physical integrity'. A degrading punishment could be inflicted both physically and mentally (anguish, fear, humiliation, feeling of inferiority). Breaking a victim's physical or moral resistance is enough to amount to degrading treatment provided the conditions of the ill-treatment are below a standard of acceptability.

Article 5 – Right to Liberty and Security   This Article covers situations of arbitrary detention, arbitrary arrest and unlawful restriction of movement. This does not mean that a person cannot be detained. However, detention must : a) be justified by public policy reasons (for instance, when restriction of liberty is the only option available to avoid a person causing harm to themselves or to third parties); and b) be carried out 'in accordance with a procedure prescribed by law' – as set out in Article 5(2) of Schedule 1. The decisions of the European Court of Human Rights indicate that the concepts of 'security of person' and 'right to liberty' are both concerned with matters of physical liberty.

Article 6 – Right to a Fair Trial   Article 6 is of significant importance in that it provides that everyone has a right to a fair judicial hearing in both criminal and civil proceedings. This Article also includes the right to challenge decisions taken outside the context of legal proceedings; for instance, the parent of a child with learning disabilities presenting severe challenging behaviours, who is placed in a special needs school, would have a right to challenge any decisions taken by the school management body, which affect that child. Article 6 not only entitles a person to be heard before a court of justice, but it also imposes an obligation on the judicial authorities to ensure that hearing procedures are conducted fairly. Article 6 states that a hearing must take place within a reasonable period of time. Furthermore, other implied rights include: that of equality between the parties; that each party is able to be physically present at the hearing to put their argument forward; to be able to bring evidence before the court or decision-making body, to summon a witness and to comment on evidence brought against them. Finally, the court is under an obligation to present a reasoned judgement.

Article 8 – Right to Respect for Private Life and Family Life   The concept of private life encapsulated in this Article implies that a person's integrity should be protected at both the physical and psychological level.

Article 10 – Freedom of Expression   The scope of Article 10 includes the right to entertain ideas and express them, as well as the right to receive information. Although there is no such right as 'freedom of information', one's right to be provided with information can nonetheless be protected by Article 10. Article 10 does not discriminate between forms of expression and covers many, such as words, pictures, paintings, images, dress and/or actions.

Article 14 – Prohibition of Discrimination   Article 14 is not actionable by itself. It can only be used in conjunction with another Convention article. For example, a person with learning disabilities, who is denied the right or opportunity to form a relationship might claim that she was being discriminated against due to having a learning disability in breach of Article 14, which prejudiced her in the exercise of her right to family life under Article 8. There is thus a breach both of her rights under Article 14, as well as under Article 8, but the discrimination alleged must be linked to the breach of the enjoyment of another right.

Article 17 – Prohibition of Abuse of Rights   It is understood that Article 17 cannot be used by itself and may only be invoked in conjunction with other Convention rights. Article 17 comes into action when a body or person attempts to evade the restrictions or guarantees (depending on the point of view) set in the Convention in a way that is not recognised or covered by the Convention. Arguably, this Article would provide a flexible safety net that would enable the courts to interpret a convention right and a violating act in the light of social changes.

Chapter 5

Case studies

Introduction

The present chapter presents case scenarios, which have been kindly provided by various sources such as care organisations (eg Voice UK), carers, parents, therapists and other professionals and bodies who wish to remain anonymous. These facts have then been followed with the advice potentially applicable in each situation.

Parental right and corporal punishment

> *Fifteen-year-old Angus, who has severe learning disabilities, has made repeated allegations that he is being beaten by his parents. Rose, his mother, admits that he is smacked as a reprimand for his behaviour. The practice of smacking is carried out with all her three children and she does not differentiate between her son with learning disabilities and her other children who do not have learning disabilities.*

Liability

Although, in England and Wales, a parent has a right to administer corporal punishment to their child, the force used must be reasonable under both criminal and civil law, Rose could be liable for assault. Under the Human Rights Act 1998, she could be in breach of Article 3, which prohibits torture and inhuman and degrading treatment and/or punishment.

Defences

Lawful Correction This defence would be available if it is proven that Rose has not used excessive force in administering the punishment to Angus and that her intention was to punish her son. If Rose inflicted a harsher punishment than a smack to Angus 'for the gratification of passion or rage', thus causing him unnecessary suffering, this would amount to assault. For a corporal chastisement to contravene Article 3 Schedule 1 Human Rights Act 1998, the force used must reach a certain degree of severity.

Reasonable Punishment The defence of reasonable punishment or lawful correction has since the implementation of Section 58 Children Act 2004 on 15 January 2005 only been available if Rose is charged with common assault. The defence will no longer be available if Rose is charged with: offences under Section 47 Offences Against the

Person Act 1861, assault occasioning actual bodily harm; offences under Section 18 or Section 20 Offences Against the Person Act 1861, wounding or causing grievous bodily harm; or an offence under Section 1 Children and Young Persons Act 1933, cruelty to persons under 16. Since 15 January 2005 in any situation in which an action might be taken in civil law for battery, Section 58(3) provides that where such battery causes actual bodily harm, then it cannot be justified in any civil proceedings on the ground that it constituted reasonable punishment.

SUMMARY ANSWER

A court of law would look at the physical and mental effect of the smack on Angus, and would also consider Angus's learning disability and his age. The English case law provides added guidance in that Angus must be able to understand the nature of the smack and the reason for the punishment. Whether in this case Rose applied a reasonable chastisement or assaulted her son it would most certainly be investigated by either the police and/or the social services, because of Angus's vulnerability and since the implementation of Section 58 Children Act 2004 on 15 January 2005 'reasonable punishment' is now only a defence to a charge of common assault and will not be available in more serious cases where the harm inflicted is more than slight and transient.

Checklist for assault and battery in Angus and Rose's case

Defences	For the defence to be successful...	YES	NO
LAWFUL CORRECTION AND REASONABLE PUNISHMENT	Does Rose have parental responsibility?	✓	
	Was the action reasonable to reprimand Angus for his behaviour?	✓	
	Was the force used reasonable and moderate, ie not excessive and not leaving any marks?	✓	
	Does Angus understand his punishment?	✓	

Physical restraint

Jack, a 12-year-old boy with autism, is living in a residential school. It is reported to his mother Mrs T. that the school has had to restrain him. His nose has been broken and there are marks where belt straps have cut into him. Jack has also made allegations that he has been held down and punched.

Liability

It is submitted that the individual members of staff could be charged with the offence of assault occasioning actual bodily harm under Section 47 Offences Against the Person Act 1861. The school may be liable in damages to Jack, for the tortious act of their employees as well damages for potential infringement of Articles 3 (prohibition of torture, inhuman and degrading treatment/punishment) and 8 (respect for private life) Schedule 1 Human Rights Act 1998.

The court would need to look at the reason why, and the circumstances in which, Jack was being restrained. However, the fact that Jack has sustained a nose injury and that the school has had to use straps to restrain him might be evidence of an excessive and possibly abusive use of force, unless a previous risk assessment of the techniques to be used when Jack needs restraining indicated the use of such straps. It should also be remembered that teachers or other members of staff at a school do not have the right to inflict corporal punishment although they are able to use appropriate restraint where the pupil may be endangering himself or others or property (see Section 131 Schools Standards and Framework Act 1998, Section 550A Education Act 1996 and see DfEE Circular on the Use of Force to Control or Restrain Pupils 10/98).

The assault might also be in direct contravention of Article 3 Human Rights Act 1998 if it is proven to be a premeditated action which has been applied for hours at a stretch and caused actual bodily injury; in particular if the suffering and humiliation endured by Jack goes beyond what is deemed to be legitimate and reasonable when administering a punishment.

The assault may also be in violation of Article 8 Human Rights Act 1998 since this article covers a person's right to physical integrity.

Defences

Necessity, if the staff had no choice but to restrain Jack in order to avoid injury to themselves or to save his life.

Self-defence, if the staff had to defend themselves against an unlawful attack from Jack.

Prevention of a breach of the peace, if Jack was a physical threat to either the staff or a third party, or threatened to damage property.

Prevention of crime, if the staff restrained Jack to prevent him from committing an offence punishable by law.

SUMMARY ANSWER

In order to avoid liability the school would need to record the incident carefully and accurately, giving all the information including the names of the staff involved, the reason for using the physical restraint, details of the risk assessment, the type of restraint employed, the date and the duration of the intervention and finally to record any injury that staff of the child might have incurred (see paragraph 11.3 DoH/DfES Guidance on the Use of Physical Interventions). This would support any plea of necessity, self-defence, prevention of a breach of the peace or prevention of a crime (assuming that Jack might have attempted to commit either) as a defence justifying their action.

Checklist for assault and battery in Jack's case

Defences	For the defences to be successful...	YES	NO
NECESSITY	Was the action necessary to save Jack's life or prevent harm occurring to him?	✓	
SELF-DEFENCE	Was the action necessary to protect the staff's own welfare and physical integrity?	✓	
PREVENTION OF A BREACH OF THE PEACE	Was the action necessary to prevent Jack being physically violent towards staff or a third party?	✓	
PREVENTION OF CRIME	Was the action necessary to stop Jack from performing an unlawful act?	✓	
ALL DEFENCES	Was the force/restraint used reasonable and necessary to avoid a greater harm from occurring?	✓	
Guidelines			
DoH/DfES GUIDANCE ON PHYSICAL INTERVENTION	Has the school made a note of the events, including all the relevant details to the restraint situation, in a record book?	✓	
DfEE GUIDANCE ON THE USE OF FORCE TO CONTROL OR RESTRAIN PUPILS	Has the school made a note of the events including all the relevant details to the restraint situation, in a record book?	✓	

Physical restraint policies

> *Damien works in a day centre for people with learning disabilities. One afternoon, 19-year-old Olivia seems agitated and upset, for no apparent reason, to the support staff, and starts kicking and punching the walls and doors, as well as throwing chairs around – no real damage could be caused since the building is designed for this kind of situation. However, the manager of the centre decides to restrain Olivia, and with the help of three other support workers holds Olivia down on the floor for 15 minutes until she calms down. Damien refuses to participate in the physical intervention as he believes that the intervention does not meet the criteria set out in the centre's policy document.*

Liability

A policy document would generally include the following sort of guidance: staff should only resort to a physical intervention after having tried first to defuse the situation; if such attempt fails, then intervention should only occur if and when a resident presents a risk or imminent danger of (a) causing physical injury to themselves, other residents or member of staff; or (b) is causing damage to property.

Failure to follow such instructions could result in liability for assault and battery, or more serious criminal offences if a resident incurs serious injuries as a consequence of the physical intervention, as well as a breach of Articles 3 (prohibition of torture and inhuman or degrading treatment/punishment), 5 (right to liberty and security) and 8 (respect for private life) Human Rights Act 1998.

Defences

Necessity/duress of circumstances, if the manager of the centre felt that the situation was such that it required immediate action and that only reasonable force was used in order to avoid a threat of injury to the staff, other residents or Olivia herself.

Consent, if Olivia has consented to that kind of intervention, ie if it has been agreed by a multi-disciplinary panel, including Olivia, that such an intervention would be part of her personal care plan.

Prevention of a breach of the peace, if Olivia's conduct would harm a third party or provoke them to respond violently or would cause damage to property.

Prevention of crime, as Olivia's conduct could be considered to be causing criminal damage to the centre's property, and could also constitute a physical threat to the health and safety of the staff and other residents if one of them should get hurt by a flying chair.

SUMMARY ANSWER

If there is a real danger that Olivia's conduct is a physical threat to herself, the staff and/or other residents, or to centre property, the staff could indeed plead necessity or duress of circumstances provided the force used is proportionate to the challenge presented by Olivia and is not excessive.

Checklist for assault and battery in Olivia's case

Defences	For the defences to be successful...	YES	NO
NECESSITY DURESS OF CIRCUMSTANCES	Was there no other alternative but for the manager of the day centre to restrain Olivia in order to avoid harm to herself, other residents or to staff happening?	✓	
CONSENT	Did Olivia agree to be restrained in order to manage her behaviour?	✓	
PREVENTION OF A BREACH OF THE PEACE	Was the action essential as Olivia's conduct posed a physical threat to staff, third parties or property?	✓	
PREVENTION OF CRIME	Was the action necessary in order to prevent Olivia from committing a criminal act?	✓	

Violence against carer

> *Twenty-five-year-old Michael, who has a learning disability, bites his carer Alan's forearm. In this situation, Alan:*
>
> *a) pinches Michael's nose in order to impede on his breathing and pull his arm out of the bite.*
> *b) forces Michael's mouth onto his forearm so as to exercise a pressure on the mouth and make the bite difficult to hold for Michael.*

Liability

Alan could be charged with assault and battery. If Michael sustains injury following the nose pinch or the pressure of Alan's forearm in his mouth, Alan could also be charged with Section 47 Offences Against the Person Act 1861 offence, and be in breach of Article 3 (prohibition of torture and inhuman or degrading treatment/punishment) of the Human Rights Act 1998.

Defences

Self-defence/necessity, as he was himself the victim of an assault and battery.

   a) On the face of it, such a defence would succeed provided the degree of force deployed by Alan is reasonable. In considering the reasonableness of Alan's reaction, it is important to bear in mind that as the support worker of a vulnerable person, he owes Michael a duty of care. For the defence to succeed, it must be an action that a reasonable person in Alan's particular circumstances – ie a support worker – would have taken.
   b) The same reasoning and principle of reasonableness apply here. It is, however, relevant to mention that forcing the forearm in the mouth in order for the bite to release the arm is likely to cause injuries such as damage to teeth, jaw, nose area, possible laceration, risk of infection if the skin is broken, and anoxia.[7]

Prevention of crime, as Michael's conduct could also constitute an assault and battery on Alan.

> **SUMMARY ANSWER**
>
> *In any court case, judges know that they have the benefit of calm consideration of circumstances after the event. They would be slow to impose liability on a person doing no more than that which he honestly thought was in the best interests of the person with severe learning disabilities presenting severe challenging behaviour.*
>
> *a) If Alan reacted instinctively and believed that pinching Michael's nose was necessary to disengage himself and if Alan did not wilfully attempt to inflict undue pain on Michael, this would be strong evidence in support of his claim of self-defence.*
> *b) It is submitted that if there are indeed other more appropriate methods of disengaging from a bite, then the defence would succeed only if these methods do not work and forcing the arm into the mouth is a last resort.*

Checklist for assault and battery in Michael's case

Defences	For the defence to be successful...	YES	NO
SELF-DEFENCE	Did Alan react instinctively to protect himself?	✓	
NECESSITY	Did Alan use what he believed was reasonable force to avoid further harm to himself?	✓	
	Did Alan only use a method that was likely to inflict the least harm possible to Michael?	✓	
PREVENTION OF CRIME	Was Alan's action necessary to stop Michael from carrying on committing an unlawful act – ie assault and battery against Alan?	✓	

Carer's liability

Jacquie, a support worker, is used as bank staff in a residential home caring for adults with learning disabilities. She is directed to do an observational session[8] with Ronan, who has cerebral palsy. Ronan is said to often become extremely upset and throw himself on the floor, flailing his arms and legs around and shouting.

Liability

If Jacquie intervenes in an attempt to prevent injury occurring to Ronan and he sustains injury, she could be charged with assault and battery. She could also possibly be liable for negligence, and in breach of Article 3 (prohibition of torture and inhuman or degrading treatment/punishment) Human Rights Act 1998.

Defences

Necessity, based on the facts as she believed them to be and on the 'best interest' principle if she believed that Ronan's physical integrity was at risk. She must show that the force she used was reasonable in the circumstances.

Mistake, if in hindsight it appears that Jacquie's intervention with Ronan was not necessary, ie if she mistakenly believed that the circumstances were such that she felt compelled to intervene.

SUMMARY ANSWER

If Jacquie genuinely intervenes with Ronan's best interest in mind and this could be proven in a court of law, it is most probable that she would avoid liability.

Checklist for negligence in Ronan's case

Defences	For the defences to be successful...	YES	NO
NECESSITY	Did Jacquie intervene in a manner that is recognised as good practice?	✓	
	Did Jacquie follow the residential home's policy guidelines for such a situation?	✓	
	Did Jacquie feel that she needed to intervene in order to either protect Ronan from hurting himself, or to prevent harm happening to her?	✓	
MISTAKE	Did Jacquie genuinely believe that an action was necessary in order to prevent harm from occurring?	✓	

Employer's liability

Daniel, a newly employed support worker in a residential home for people with learning disabilities, clearly indicates to the care manager that he is not trained in physical intervention techniques. He asks for support guidelines on manual handling concerning certain residents who are known to present severe challenging behaviours which might require a physical intervention. The only verbal instruction given to him is to stay away if and when such a situation occurs, and to call for help if necessary.

Liability

If Daniel sustains injury following an intervention, the residential home might be liable for failure to provide Daniel with a safe place and system of work, which could include the duty to provide training in physical intervention techniques.

If Daniel follows the care manager's instructions, he would not be personally liable for omitting to act. However, the residential home (represented by the care manager), as Daniel's employer, would be vicariously liable for any injury sustained by a resident as a result of Daniel's omission to act. Although an omission in itself would not give rise to liability, in a situation where there is a contractual duty to act or a special relationship between the parties, as is the case between a care staff employer and the residents, the courts might find that there is a breach of duty. The residential home has a duty of care towards the residents and could thus be held vicariously liable in negligence. In a situation where Daniel disregarded the care manager's instructions and a resident incurred an injury as a result of Daniel's physical intervention, the residential home could also be held vicariously liable for the physical intervention performed by Daniel even if the intervention was wrongfully performed and despite the fact that it was forbidden by the care manager.

Defence to an action brought by Daniel against the home

No breach of duty of care/standard of care. Again, this is not a defence *per se*. However, if the home can prove that all reasonable steps were taken to ensure that Daniel is provided with a safe place and system of work, which is in accordance with the general practice in this field, there would be no liability for negligence.

Defences to actions against the home

No breach of duty of care/standard of care. Although this is not a defence *per se*, if the residential home could prove that there is no breach of duty, there would be no liability for negligence. Thus, if it can be proven that a responsible body of skilled professionals, would find the practice deployed by the residential home as proper, even if it can also be argued that a body of opinion would suggest the use of a different technique, then the home could escape liability in negligence.

Necessity, if Daniel had to intervene in order to prevent harm from happening to himself, a resident or a third party, or to prevent a resident from causing damage to property.

Self-defence, if Daniel, fearing for his personal safety, had to defend himself, or another person to whom he owes a duty of care, against a physical attack from a resident.

Prevention of a breach of the peace, if Daniel felt that he should intervene in order to prevent a resident from breaking the peace in the residential home, which could worsen a situation and possibly endanger the rest of the residents, staff and other third parties such as members of the public visiting the premises within the walls of the residence at the time of the challenging situation arising.

Prevention of crime, if Daniel could not do otherwise but to restrain a resident to prevent the latter committing a crime.

SUMMARY ANSWER

For a claim in negligence to succeed, it must be established that the residential home owes a duty of care towards its residents and that that duty has been breached. Although residents might suffer harm as a result of physical intervention performed by the residential home's staff, if it is proven that this kind of intervention is recognised as good practice by a responsible body of fellow professionals, it is argued that the residential home would not be in breach of a duty of care and would thus avoid liability in negligence.

Checklist for duty of care in the residential home's case

Defences	For the defences to be successful...	YES	NO
STANDARD OF CARE – AS REGARDS DANIEL	Were all the reasonable measures taken to ensure Daniel's health and safety?	✓	
DUTY OF CARE – AS REGARDS THE RESIDENTS	Was Daniel's intervention within the ambit of the residential home's appropriate and reasonable care provided to its residents?	✓	
NECESSITY	Was Daniel's action essential to prevent harm happening to himself or the residents?	✓	
SELF-DEFENCE	Did he need to protect and defend himself from a resident's actions?	✓	
PREVENTION OF A BREACH OF THE PEACE	Was an action required to prevent a violent incident from happening in the residential home, in which other residents, staff or visitors could be harmed?	✓	
PREVENTION OF CRIME	Did Daniel stop a resident committing an unlawful act?	✓	

Incident recording

> *Jo, a 10-year-old boy with autism living in a residential special school, has sustained a number of physical injuries and bruising over a period of two years, some of which were accounted for and others that were unexplained. His mother has made formal complaints to the local authority that placed her son and to the local authority where the child resides.*

Liability

If Jo has presented the staff with challenging situations which has led them to use physical interventions on him, and he has been physically marked by these interventions, this would suggest that he was the victim of assault and battery. There would also appear to be a breach of some of his Convention rights, namely Article 3 (prohibition of torture and inhuman or degrading treatment/punishment), Article 5 (right to liberty and security) and Article 8 (right to respect for private life and family life) Human Rights Act 1998 as well as a breach of Section 175 Education Act 2002 which now provides that it is the duty of the school and the governing body to safeguard and promote the welfare of the child while he is in school. If the school is a privately run school, it will be subject to identical regulation by Section 157 of the Education Act 2002.

Under Section 131 Schools Standards and Framework Act 1998, school staff have no right to administer corporal punishment to pupils.

If, after investigation, it appears that Jo has been physically abused by members of staff, the local authority would be held in breach of a duty of care. The local authority would be held vicariously liable for failing to take reasonable steps to protect and safeguard Jo in his physical, moral and educational development at the school.

If on the contrary, Jo has been bullied at the school, the local authority could be held to be in breach of its duty of care for failing to take appropriate steps to stop the bullying under the provisions of Section 61(4)(b) Schools Standards and Framework Act 1998, and again in breach of the provisions of Section 175 or Section 157 of the Education Act 2002.

Defences

Lawful excuse, which could be supported by recording the incident in an incident book as this is not only a duty but could also serve as proof in case of a criminal charge or civil liability. The lawful excuse could be necessity, self-defence, duress of circumstances and/or illegality.

Prevention of a breach of the peace, assuming the staff felt they had to intervene, as Jo's conduct was a threat to himself, the staff and/or other people or property in his vicinity.

Prevention of crime, if the staff had to intervene in order to prevent Jo from committing an unlawful act.

SUMMARY ANSWER

Paragraph 11.3 DoH/DfES Guidance on the Use of Physical Interventions says that whether they are planned or unplanned, these physical interventions 'should always be recorded as quickly as practicable (in any event within 24 hours of the incident) by the person(s) involved in the incident in a book with numbered pages'. The latter would provide the local authority with a possible defence/lawful excuse that would justify a physical intervention upon Jo.

Checklist for assault and battery in Jo's case

Defences	For the defences to be successful...	YES	NO
LAWFUL EXCUSE	Was the physical intervention the only remedy available to deal with Jo's behaviour?	✓	
	Was the force used reasonable?	✓	
	Was the force excessive – ie are there any visible physical marks, bruises, cuts as a result of the physical intervention?		✗
PREVENTION OF A BREACH OF THE PEACE	Was Jo's conduct a physical threat to other pupils or staff, or was likely to damage property?	✓	
PREVENTION OF CRIME	Was Jo's conduct of a criminal nature?	✓	

Guidelines

DoH/DfES GUIDANCE ON PHYSICAL INTERVENTION	Has a record of the event been kept in the record book?	✓
GUIDANCE ON SAFEGUARDING CHILDREN IN EDUCATION	Has there been compliance with Circular 0027/2004 Safeguarding Children in Education and Further Education Institutes (DfES 2004)	✓

Medical treatment and liability

> *Twenty-two-year-old Lorna has a learning disability and mental illness and refuses to eat because she says to Marie, her key worker, that it is the only way she can exercise some control over her general behaviour. An assessment has shown that for her, it is a form of either prevention or punishment for acting in a particular way.*

Liability

On the one hand, Marie, Lorna's key worker, owes her a duty of care due to their special relationship. An omission to act in these circumstances would most likely lead Lorna to starve to death and could thus be held to be negligent and in violation of Article 2 (right to life) Human Rights Act 1998. On the other hand, if Marie decides to intervene and administer a treatment to Lorna against her will, despite the fact that it would protect and maintain her health and life, Marie could face a charge of assault and battery.

Defences

Necessity, as an omission to intervene would imply that Marie is 'assisting' Lorna in her suicide attempt.

Consent, which could come in the form of a court order allowing her to try and feed Lorna, even though it is against the latter's will.

> **SUMMARY ANSWER**
>
> *Before administering the treatment to Lorna, Marie must first seek to obtain a court order rendering the proposed treatment lawful. The court is likely to overrule Lorna's refusal to consent to treatment since it would be in her best interest to save her life. This position would be the same if Lorna was a minor. Furthermore, Article 2 (right to life) of the Human Rights Act 1998 cannot be interpreted as conferring a right to die, nor does it create 'a right to self-determination' that would entitle Lorna to choose death over life.*

Checklist for assault and battery in Lorna's case

Defences	For the defences to be successful...	YES	NO
CONSENT	Has Marie sought a court order to override Lorna's refusal to eat?	✓	
NECESSITY	Was Marie's action necessary in order to save Lorna's life?	✓	
	Is it in Lorna's best interest that she should receive the appropriate medical treatment to remedy her refusal to feed herself without her consent?	✓	

Medical treatment and consent

> Dr Jones is a general practitioner and deals with many patients who have learning disabilities and severely challenging behaviour. He is sometimes called upon to administer certain medication to his patients either as part of a long-term treatment programme or as an emergency measure in order to deal with the patients' challenging behaviours. He is concerned about his potential liabilities, in particular as regards the issue of consent to medical treatment.

Liability

If Dr Jones administers medication without his patients' consent, and/or without the consent of a person who could do so on behalf of his patients, he could be facing liability in negligence, as well as a charge for assault and battery. He could also be in breach of Article 3 (prohibition of torture and inhuman or degrading treatment/punishment), Article 5 (right to liberty and security), Article 8 (right to respect for private life and family life) and Article 10 (freedom of expression) Human Rights Act 1998.

When seeking consent from his patients, Dr Jones must ensure that his patients: a) have the capacity to give consent; b) are informed as to the nature, purpose, potential risks and consequences of the proposed treatments, as well as to any alternative therapeutic methods available; and c) give their consent freely and voluntarily.

Where Dr Jones's patients are children, he can also seek consent from them, provided they have a sufficient understanding and intelligence to give consent; or from their parents or someone who has parental responsibility. 'Understanding' means an under-standing of the treatment, its purpose, benefits and risks, and the consequences of not receiving such treatment. It also means that the child has capacity for making a choice.

Defences

Necessity or duress of circumstances, in case of an emergency intervention, these defences could be pleaded if the medical intervention is in the patient's best interests, ie necessary to save his life or avoid physical injury; or when it is necessary in order to prevent a third party, or the GP himself being hurt by the patient. Treatment can also be given without consent if it is necessary to alleviate a disorder or prevent deterioration of the patient's condition in the long term.

Consent would justify and make legal Dr Jones's medical intervention either in an emergency situation, or as part of a long-term medical treatment programme.

Prevention of a breach of the peace, if Dr Jones feels that a medical intervention is necessary if a patient presents a physical threat him (Dr Jones) or a third party.

Prevention of crime, if a patient is about to commit a crime and can only be prevented from doing so by being given a medical intervention that would restrain them from acting unlawfully.

SUMMARY ANSWER

Dr Jones would not be acting unlawfully if he obtained consent before administering medical treatment, or if he acted out of necessity in an emergency situation to protect either the patient engaging in the behaviour, or to protect any other patients, members of staff, or visitors to the home. In any given circumstances, when consent is not given, treatment should only be given in the interests of the patient and not the carer.

Checklist for assault and battery in Dr Jones's patients' case

Defences	For the defences to be successful...	YES	NO
NECESSITY/ DURESS OF CIRCUMSTANCES	Does an emergency require that medical intervention be administered by Dr Jones?	✓	
	Is such a measure in the best interest of the patient?	✓	
	Is it a reasonable and least harmful method?	✓	
CONSENT	Has Dr Jones been given consent to proceed with a medical intervention?	✓	
	Has consent been given by the patient or a legal representative of the patient?	✓	
	Was it an informed consent?	✓	
PREVENTION OF A BREACH OF THE PEACE	Is medical intervention necessary to prevent a patient from being a physical threat to the GP or third parties?	✓	
PREVENTION OF CRIME	Does Dr Jones need to intervene to prevent a criminal act being carried out by a patient?	✓	

Therapeutic treatment and assault

Colin, an eight-year-old boy with cerebral palsy affecting mainly his legs, has a home programme, performed by his father, which includes the use of some firm pressure to maintain the ranges of movement in the child's ankle joint to prevent further deformity and loss of function and also some difficult exercises. The challenge and difficulty of the therapy programme for the child has been explained by the therapist and the need for gentle encouragement over time has been emphasised. However, at the next appointment Colin's father says that the child is lazy and cries at anything and has to be pushed all the time. He reports that he makes the child do the exercises until he (the father) is satisfied. The father tells the therapist that she is too soft and he knows his child best.

Liability

Although the exercises appear to be in Colin's best interests, pushing him to perform them until his father is satisfied to the point where Colin cries due to pain clearly is not.

This could amount to assault in that the father demonstrates an intention to force Colin to carry on with the exercises despite his discomfort and pain. This could also qualify as a violation of Colin's right not to be subjected to inhuman and degrading treatment, under Article 3 (prohibition of torture and inhuman or degrading treatment/punishment) Schedule 1 Human Rights Act 1998.

It is argued that Colin is being exposed to undue and unnecessary suffering, causing him 'significant harm', which, under Section 31 Children Act 1989, would mean that he is suffering from ill-treatment or an impairment of his health and development.

It could also be argued that the State is in breach of Article 3 of the Human Rights Act 1998 in failing to protect Colin from his father's conduct.

Defences

Lawful correction, provided it is proven that the father's behaviour does not threaten Colin's life and integrity of limbs and that his perseverance is not for his own satisfaction but is actually in the best interests of the child and since implementation of the Children Act 2004, Section 58 on 15 January 2005 the defence of reasonable punishment can only be used in respect of a charge of common assault and not to a charge of cruelty under Section 1 Children and Young Persons Act 1933.

Necessity, which can justify the attitude of Colin's father as the programme is a necessary process that will help improve Colin's quality of life in the longer-term. This also comes under the issue of medical treatment and consent. If it can be proved that the father's perseverance is deemed reasonable, that he is not inflicting unnecessary suffering upon his son, then the defence of necessity could be raised.

SUMMARY ANSWER

Colin's father could rely on paragraph 8.1 of the DoH/DfES Guidance on the Use of Physical Interventions, which provides: 'occasionally, it may be considered in the best interests of the child or adult to accept the possible use of restrictive physical intervention as part of a therapeutic or educational strategy that could not be introduced without accepting that reasonable force might be required.'

Checklist for assault and battery in Colin's case

Defences	For the defence to be successful...	YES	NO
LAWFUL CORRECTION	Is the father's conduct in the best interest of Colin?	✓	
	Is the degree of force in the intervention reasonable?	✓	
NECESSITY	Is Colin subjected to unnecessary suffering?		✗
	Is the programme essential to better Colin's quality of life?	✓	

Physical restraint for therapeutic purposes and false imprisonment

Liability

The parents of Dennis, a five-year-old-boy with epilepsy and cerebral palsy and whose hips are being monitored for potential risks of dislocation, ask the physiotherapist for some night time splinting for their son. The parents say that such splinting is essential to prevent their son's hip position deteriorating. Previously the mother had asked the physiotherapist for a bed with high sides because the child would not stay in bed at night. This had been declined because there was no therapeutic indication for this. Advice had been given on making the bedroom environment safe and a stair gate was in place at home.

It would appear that the motive for Dennis's parents' request for splinting is either to restrict his movement at night time, or to help prevent a hip dislocation. They could face a charge of false imprisonment for the use of a bed with high sides, or for false imprisonment and battery for the use of splinting. Dennis's parents could also be in violation of Article 3 (prohibition of torture and inhuman or degrading treatment/punishment), Article 5 (right to liberty and security) and Article 8 (right to respect for private life and family life) Human Rights Act 1998.

The DoH/DfES guidance on physical interventions provides that any devices usually used for therapeutic purposes cannot be used as a method of behaviour control.

Defences

Lawful Correction, provided the physical intervention is deemed reasonable and does not impose unnecessary suffering on Dennis, and if his parents fear that Dennis would injure himself during the night if his mobility was not restricted.

Necessity, if it can be medically proven that the splinting would prevent Dennis from dislocating his hip. It could thus be said that the splinting is for therapeutic use and as such would be in the child's best interests. It could also be justified on this basis if Dennis's parents have no other choice than to use physical restrictions in order to avoid Dennis from getting injured during the night, when they cannot watch him every hour.

SUMMARY ANSWER

If Dennis' parents can argue and bring evidence that Dennis is at risk of significant harm at night time, that the therapist's suggestions to make the bedroom safer have failed, then paragraph 5.3 of the DoH/DfES Guidance on the Use of Physical Interventions *provides that 'a decision to use therapeutic devices to prevent problem behaviour must be agreed by a multi-disciplinary team in consultation with service users, their families and advocates (...)'. It is submitted that the therapist cannot simply dismiss the child's parents' concerns. They would have a right to be heard and have their case properly assessed and eventually discussed in a multi-disciplinary meeting.*

Checklist for false imprisonment in Dennis's case

Defences	For the defences to be successful...	YES	NO
LAWFUL CORRECTION	Is the action reasonable, ie not excessive?	✓	
	Does Dennis incur unnecessary suffering?		✗
NECESSITY	Is the splitting essential, as the only viable option, to prevent Dennis incurring harm?	✓	
	Is the intervention in Dennis' best interest?	✓	

False imprisonment and seclusion

Liability

Thirty-two-year-old Joanne, who has an autistic spectrum disorder, recently moved into a residential home. When she is upset, she starts attacking people around her, trying to kick them. Physical restraint, such as trying to hold her, only stimulates her more, leading her to start screaming. After making some observations and assessing the risks posed by other measures, the staff came to the conclusion that seclusion works better for Joanne as she would calm down easily and more rapidly.

This method, however successful, cannot be inserted into an individual care plan as part of a treatment programme as it is an emergency method – only to be used as a last resort for the shortest time possible. The staff could face a charge for false imprisonment and be in breach of Article 3 (prohibition of torture and inhuman or degrading treatment/punishment), Article 5 (right to liberty and security) and Article 8 (right to respect for private life and family life) Human Rights Act 1998.

Defences

Necessity/duress of circumstances, if the staff have no other choice but to isolate Joanne as she presents a physical threat to other people around her. This would be particularly valid as holding Joanne would most likely worsen the situation.

Consent, if Joanne consents to be taken away and isolated from the rest of the people around her during an intervention where she attempts to hurt someone else.

SUMMARY ANSWER

It could be argued that Joanne calms down when she is moved into another environment, possibly where she is alone and has no other stimuli to upset her. In this context, moving Joanne into another room or another area of the residence would be an appropriate measure provided all appropriate measures are taken to ensure Joanne's safety and protection. It would allow Joanne time and space to deal with her emotions and inner conflicts. However, Joanne should never be put into a locked room, as this would amount to false imprisonment.

Checklist for false imprisonment in Joanne's case

Defences	For the defence to be successful...	YES	NO
NECESITY DURESS OF CIRCUMSTANCES	Is the action necessary to prevent Joanne causing harm to third parties?	✓	
	Is the action the least harmful and in Joanne's best interests?	✓	
CONSENT	Has Joanne given her consent to be led to another area when she starts attacking people?	✓	
	Joanne is not led into a restrictive area where doors are locked, or from where she cannot leave at free will.		✗

False imprisonment and locking

Chloë is a citizen advocate who visits residents in care homes for people with learning disabilities who also present severe challenging behaviours. She has observed that most care homes have locked doors that are opened through a buzzer system activated when a person presses on a button to go through the doors. A member of staff stationed in the entrance booth allows the opening of the door after checking who buzzes. Residents and visitors can neither enter nor exit the care home without being buzzed in or out by the staff in the entrance booth. Chloë wonders about the legality of such a system.

Liability

Prima facie, the care home could be liable for false imprisonment, as the buzzing system appears to restrict residents' freedom of movement, and would thus be in breach of Article 5 (Right to Liberty and Security) and possibly Article 8 (Right to Respect for Private Life and Family Life) Schedule 1 Human Rights Act 1998.

Defences

Necessity, if it is necessary for the residents, staff and visitors' physical health and safety that the residents are not allowed to move about freely.

Common law/statutory power to detain the insane, if the residents are described as 'insane' and are considered to be likely 'to do mischief to [themselves] or any other person'.

Prevention of a breach of the peace, if the residents are a physical threat to each other, members of staff and/or visitors, or property.

Prevention of crime, if the locking system is necessary in order to prevent crimes being committed if residents were allowed to go through the doors unchecked.

SUMMARY ANSWER

Locking the doors through a buzzer system may not necessarily be illegal, as it can be seen as a reasonable measure that is necessary for the safeguard of the care home's residents, staff and visitors. However, it could constitute a false imprisonment if the buzzer system is solely used for the staff's own benefit, that is unrelated to their physical health, but only to facilitate their duties. Locking doors for that reason cannot justify the violation of residents' freedom of movement.

Checklist for false Imprisonment in Chloë's case

Defences	For the defences to be successful...	YES	NO
NECESSITY	Is the action necessary to ensure residents, visitors and staff's health and safety?	✓	
POWER TO DETAIN THE INSANE	Are the residents and visitors at risk of coming to harm without the measure?	✓	
PREVENTION OF A BREACH OF THE PEACE	Do the residents represent a physical threat to each other, visitors and/or staff?	✓	
PREVENTION OF CRIME	Is the action essential to prevent criminal conduct occurring?	✓	

Appendix

Human rights law – relevant articles

Article 2 – Right to life

1. Everyone's right to life shall be protected by law. No one shall be deprived of his life intentionally save in the execution of a sentence of a court following his conviction of a crime for which this penalty is provided by law.

2. Deprivation of life shall not be regarded as inflicted in contravention of this Article when it results from the use of force which is no more than absolutely necessary:

   (a) in defence of any person from unlawful violence;

   (b) in order to effect a lawful arrest or to prevent the escape of a person lawfully detained;

   (c) in action lawfully taken for the purpose of quelling a riot or insurrection.

Article 3 – Prohibition of torture and inhuman or degrading treatment

No one shall be subjected to torture or to inhuman or degrading treatment or punishment.

Article 5 – Right to liberty and security

1. Everyone has the right to liberty and security of person. No one shall be deprived of his liberty save in the following cases and in accordance with a procedure prescribed by law:

   (a) the lawful detention of a person after conviction by a competent court;

   (b) the lawful arrest or detention of a person for non-compliance with the lawful order of a court or in order to secure the fulfilment of any obligation prescribed by law;

   (c) the lawful arrest or detention of a person effected for the purpose of bringing him before the competent legal authority on reasonable suspicion of having committed an offence or when it is reasonably considered necessary to prevent his committing an offence or fleeing after having done so;

(d) the detention of a minor by lawful order for the purpose of educational supervision or his lawful detention for the purpose of bringing him before the competent legal authority;

(e) the lawful detention of persons for the prevention of the spreading of infectious diseases, of persons of unsound mind, alcoholics or drug addicts or vagrants;

(f) the lawful arrest or detention of a person to prevent his effecting an unauthorised entry into the country or of a person against whom action is being taken with a view to deportation or extradition.

2. Everyone who is arrested shall be informed promptly, in a language which he understands, of the reasons for his arrest and of any charge against him.

3. Everyone arrested or detained in accordance with the provisions of paragraph 1(c) of this Article shall be brought promptly before a judge or other officer authorised by law to exercise judicial power and shall be entitled to trial within a reasonable time or to release pending trial. Release may be conditioned by guarantees to appear for trial.

4. Everyone who is deprived of his liberty by arrest or detention shall be entitled to take proceedings by which the lawfulness of his detention shall be decided speedily by a court and his release ordered if the detention is not lawful.

5. Everyone who has been the victim of arrest or detention in contravention of the provisions of this Article shall have an enforceable right to compensation.

Article 6 – Right to a fair trial

1. In the determination of his civil rights and obligations or of any criminal charge against him, everyone is entitled to a fair and public hearing within a reasonable time by an independent and impartial tribunal established by law. Judgment shall be pronounced publicly but the press and public may be excluded from all or part of the trial in the interest of morals, public order or national security in a democratic society, where the interests of juveniles or the protection of the private life of the parties so require, or to the extent strictly necessary in the opinion of the court in special circumstances where publicity would prejudice the interests of justice.

2. Everyone charged with a criminal offence shall be presumed innocent until proved guilty according to law.

3. Everyone charged with a criminal offence has the following minimum rights:

a) to be informed promptly, in a language which he understands and in detail, of the nature and cause of the accusation against him;

b) to have adequate time and facilities for the preparation of his defence;

c) to defend himself in person or through legal assistance of his own choosing or, if he has not sufficient means to pay for legal assistance, to be given it free when the interests of justice so require;

d) to examine or have examined witnesses against him and to obtain the attendance and examination of witnesses on his behalf under the same conditions as witnesses against him;

e) to have the free assistance of an interpreter if he cannot understand or speak the language used in court.

Article 8 – Right to respect for private life and family life

1. Everyone has the right to respect for his private and family life, his home and his correspondence.

2. There shall be no interference by a public authority with the exercise of this right except such as is in accordance with the law and is necessary in a democratic society in the interests of national security, public safety or the economic well-being of the country, for the prevention of disorder or crime, for the protection of health or morals, or for the protection of the rights and freedoms of others.

Article 10 – Freedom of expression

1. Everyone has the right to freedom of expression. This right shall include freedom to hold opinions and to receive and impart information and ideas without interference by public authority and regardless of frontiers. This Article shall not prevent States from requiring the licensing of broadcasting, television or cinema enterprises.

2. The exercise of these freedoms, since it carries with it duties and responsibilities, may be subject to such formalities, conditions, restrictions or penalties as are prescribed by law and are necessary in a democratic society, in the interests of national security, territorial integrity or public safety, for the prevention of disorder or crime, for the protection of health or morals, for the protection of the reputation or rights of others, for preventing the disclosure of information received in confidence, or for maintaining the authority and impartiality of the judiciary.

Article 14 – Prohibition of discrimination

The enjoyment of the rights and freedoms set forth in this Convention shall be secured without discrimination on any ground such as sex, race, colour, language, religion, political or other opinion, national or social origin, association with a national minority, property, birth or other status.

Article 17 – Prohibition of abuse of rights

Nothing in this Convention may be interpreted as implying for any State, group or person any right to engage in any activity or perform any act aimed at the destruction of any of the rights and freedoms set forth herein or at their limitation to a greater extent than is provided for in the Convention.

Index of definitions

Definitions

Abuse

The notion of abuse is defined in the DoH guidance *No Secrets* as 'a violation of an individual's human and civil rights by any other person or persons.'[9]

Adult

Although there is no specific statutory definition of this term, the Family Law Reform Act 1969 (implemented in 1971) provided for England and Wales that the age of majority be reduced from twenty one to eighteen. Section 1(1) of that Act provides that a person attains 'full age' on attaining the age of eighteen instead of, as formerly, on attaining the age of twenty one.

Capacity

Under the criminal law, there is a presumption in England and Wales that a person aged ten or over is capable of committing a crime unless there is evidence to show that the person lacks mental capacity due to disability or mental illness. Under the law of torts, (see civil law) there is no defence of minority available to children. A child could therefore be sued in tort but in reality it rarely happens as the child will usually have no money to satisfy a judgement for damages.

In relation to medical treatment, capacity is the right to express one's mind by determining what is the best or chosen course of action to be taken in a given situation. The concept of capacity implies that a person has the ability to:

- comprehend the nature of their condition and the proposed treatment;

- understand the information and the possible consequences of consenting or not to such a treatment, in terms of the principal benefits and risks;

- make a decision based on the understanding of the information provided.

The level of capacity required depends on the seriousness or gravity of the decision which needs to be taken, and so capacity is reviewed on an individual case-by-case basis.

In relation to mental capacity the basic principles are laid out in paragraph 15.10 of the Mental Health Act 1983 'Code of Practice' and broadly cover the same issues as those outlined above. Note any new Mental Capacity legislation may affect this area.

Carer

A **parent carer** is a parent who cares for his or her disabled child.[10] Under Section 2(9) Children Act 1989, a person with parental responsibility may arrange for some or all of this responsibility to be met by one or more persons on his or her behalf. Thus, the carer does not have parental responsibility as such, although the parent has delegated some aspects relating to the care, control and safety of his or her child to the carer.

A **carer, other than a parent or other person with parental responsibility**, is a person who is involved in providing for the care, control and safety of children, young people and adults with learning disabilities presenting severe challenging behaviour. 'Carer' could include day centre workers, childminders, teachers, residential workers, respite carers, health workers, employees of voluntary organisations and of local authority social services departments.

An **unpaid carer** is someone who has not entered into a contract to care for another person. The unpaid carer is described as someone who looks after 'a relative or friend who needs support because of age, physical or learning disability or illness, including mental illness'.[11]

A **care worker** is defined in Section 80(2) of the Care Standards Act 2000 as:

'(a) an individual who is or has been employed in a position which is such as to enable him to have regular contact in the course of his duties with adults to whom accommodation is provided at a care home;

(b) an individual who is or has been employed in a position which is such as to enable him to have regular contact in the course of his duties with adults to whom prescribed services are provided by an independent hospital, an independent clinic, an independent medical agency or a National Health Service body;

(c) an individual who is or has been employed in a position which is concerned with the provision of personal care in their own homes for persons who by reason of illness, infirmity or disability are unable to provide it for themselves without assistance.'

A **care provider for adults** is defined in Section 80(7) Care Standards Act 2000 as:

(a) any person who carries on a care home;

(b) any person who carries on a domiciliary care agency;

(c) any person who carries on an independent hospital, an independent clinic or an independent medical agency, which provides prescribed services; and

(d) a National Health Service body which provides prescribed services.'

Responsibilities of carers and local authorities

Carers in general

The Department of Health White Paper, *Valuing People*, sets out four key principles in a programme to help improve, safeguard and guarantee the rights of children, young people and adults with learning disabilities, which are: rights, independence, choice and inclusion.[12]

Rights: 'People with learning disabilities have the right to a decent education, to grow up to vote, to marry and have a family, and to express their opinions, with help and support to do so where necessary.' The overall aim is to ensure the promotion and safeguarding of people with learning disabilities' civil and legal rights and to eradicate social discrimination.

Independence: '. . . while people's individual needs will differ, the starting presumption should be one of independence, rather than dependence, with public services providing the support needed to maximise this. Independence in this context does not mean doing everything unaided.'

Choice: '. . . everyone should be able to make choices. This includes people with severe and profound disabilities who, with the right help and support, can make important choices and express preferences about their day to day lives.'

Inclusion: '. . . inclusion means enabling people with learning disabilities to do. . . ordinary things, make use of mainstream services and be fully included in the local community.'

As part of the Government's objectives, carers and local authorities have a responsibility a) to increase and promote disabled children's chances to benefit from adequate educational, social and health care; and b) to enable people with learning disabilities to reach a certain level of independence and autonomy which would allow them more control over their own day-to-day lives, including the planning of their person-centred care plan.

Furthermore, carers should benefit from help and support from all relevant 'local agencies in order to fulfil their family and caring roles effectively'. In addition, such unpaid carers have an entitlement to the assessment of their needs for care or the provision of services themselves under the terms of the Carers (Recognition and Services Act 1995). Alternatively, the assessment under Section 1(2) of the Act might conclude that they are not fit themselves to take on such burdensome responsibilities and that the person for whom they are caring must be provided instead with services under the National Health Service and Community Care Act 1990.

Carers who look after children and young people

A local authority has certain rights and duties towards carers of disabled children. Section 2(1) Carers and Disabled Children Act 2000 provides that:

> *'the local authority must consider the assessment and decide a) whether the carer has needs in relation to the care which he provides or intends to*

provide; b) if so, whether they could be satisfied (wholly or partly) by services which the local authority may provide; and c) if they could be so satisfied, whether or not to provide services to the carer'.

Those carers over the age of 16 looking after children, in whatever context, would be expected to do all that is necessary to prevent the child harming him/herself or others, or exposing him/herself or others to harm with due respect to the child's functional ability rather than chronological age. (Statutory authority for this duty of care can be found in Section 1 Children and Young Persons Act 1933, which provides for the imposition of criminal liability on parents or those over 16 looking after children who fail to protect them from ill treatment, neglect or abuse; and Section 3(5) Children Act 1989, which provides for the civil standard of care, which if breached could, under the provisions of Section 31 Children Act 1989, result in the removal of the child from wherever she is being cared for and the possible institution of care proceedings on the basis that the child 'is suffering or likely to suffer significant harm').

Very importantly, Section 3(5)(a) and (b) provide that: 'A person who does not have parental responsibility for a particular child may (subject to the provisions of this Act) do what is reasonable in all circumstances of the case for the purpose of safeguarding or promoting the child's welfare'.

Challenging behaviour and severely challenging behaviour

The term 'challenging behaviour' is used in an attempt to designate an individual's behaviour which represents a 'challenge' to themselves, their environment (both people and property) and/or society in general. Such behaviour may be classified as 'seriously challenging' where there is perceived to be a greater risk of the individual's behaviour potentially harming himself, others, or damaging property, or where it is perceived as representing a greater challenge to the capacities of those who have to deal with both the behaviour and its consequences. The use of such terms, however, does not refer to an intrinsic 'wrongness' with the person presenting the challenge, but is rather reflective of a situation which is defined and interpreted by social factors.

Emerson et al (1987) defined severe challenging behaviour in the Mansell Report (1993) as:

> *'behaviour of such intensity, frequency or duration that the physical safety of the person or others is placed in serious jeopardy or behaviour which is likely to seriously limit or deny access to the use of community facilities. Ordinarily it would be expected that the person would have shown the pattern of behaviour that presents such a challenge to services for a considerable period of time. Severely challenging behaviour is not a transient phenomenon.'*

This was modified by Emerson in 1995, when he defined challenging behaviour as:

> *'culturally abnormal behaviours of such an intensity, frequency or duration that the physical safety of the person or others is likely to be placed in serious jeopardy, or behaviour which is likely to seriously limit use of, or result in the person being denied, ordinary access to ordinary community services.'*[13]

The Committee on Services for Children with a Learning Disability and Severely Challenging Behaviour, established by the Mental Health Foundation in 1993 and which finally reported in 1997,[14] adopted a rather more expanded working definition of severely challenging behaviour, which many of those working in the field found more acceptable. Thus, this Committee defined severely challenging behaviour as:

> *'Behaviour of such an intensity, frequency, or duration that the physical safety of the person or others is likely to be placed in serious jeopardy, or behaviour which is likely to seriously limit or deny access to and use of ordinary community facilities or impair a child's personal growth, development and family life. It should be emphasised that such behaviour represents a challenge to services and that definitions are therefore based on social judgements (what challenges one service or institution may not challenge another) and definitions must be considered in context.'*

The authors of this guide consider that a challenging behaviour can be more precisely or particularly described by the actual forms it can take – in other words, a challenging behaviour is arguably situation-based and socially-defined.

Child

The law in England and Wales adopts an essentially chronological approach to the definition of 'child'. Thus, in English and Welsh civil law, when the term 'child' is used it is either used specifically to denote the legal capacities attributable to such a person or to denote a relationship between two persons. For the purposes of this guide, therefore, the definition adopted in the Children Act 1989 has been used. Section 105(1) of the Children Act 1989 defines a child as being 'a person under the age of 18'.

Child in need

Section 17 Children Act (1989) defines a 'child in need' as a child who is:

● unlikely to achieve or maintain, or to have the opportunity of achieving or maintaining, a reasonable standard of health or development without the provision for him of services by a local authority, or

● his health or development is likely to be significantly impaired or further impaired without the provision for him of such services, or

● he is disabled.

Sections 17A and 17B Children Act 1989 make special provision for the making of direct payments to cover the provision of services to parents looking after disabled children, to disabled young people themselves of 16 and 17, and to any disabled person with parental responsibility for a child, where the individual wishes to choose for themselves the providers of such services to the child in need.

Civil law

The civil law in England and Wales is concerned with the regulation of conduct between legal individuals (which may include companies or government departments as well as individual people), on a one-to-one basis and encompasses many areas.

The law of torts as well as aspects of employment law and family law are parts of civil law of particular relevance to this work. Tort law requires that if any person is aggrieved or injured by the conduct of another, then they must individually take action against that other person in respect of the civil wrong (usually referred to by lawyers as a 'tort') which the conduct discloses. A tort is defined as 'a wrongful act or omission for which damages can be obtained in a civil court by the person wronged'.[15]

For example, the tort of negligence is concerned with civil law actions between legal individuals. Under the tort of negligence, assuming that there is proof of the existence of a duty of care between the two individuals, the breach of such duty by one of them (the wrongdoer, referred to in legal terms as the 'tortfeasor') will entitle the other (the individual who has suffered the wrongdoing referred to in legal terms as the 'plaintiff') to bring an action against the other for damages (ie monetary compensation). Damages, however, are not the only remedy available. Depending on the issue, a plaintiff may ask for an injunction, which is an order of the court forbidding the tortfeasor from acting in a certain manner or ordering him to perform a certain act so as to avoid or prevent harm from happening to the plaintiff.

The same circumstances which give rise to the possible prosecution of an individual under the criminal law may also amount to the commission of a civil wrong. This means that an offender can be charged by the Police and prosecuted by the Crown Prosecution Service, and may also be sued by his victim in a civil court of law. An offender can thus be convicted in the criminal court for assault and battery, and may also have to pay civil law damages to the victim in reparation for the injury that the latter has incurred. However, a civil claim for damages does not necessarily depend on a criminal conviction to succeed. Indeed, a civil action can still be brought against an offender even though the act causing the injury may not be so serious as to amount to a criminal offence, which would thus lead the Crown Prosecution Service not to pursue the matter before a court of criminal law.

The torts of particular potential relevance to those caring for adults and children with challenging behaviour include: assault, battery, false imprisonment and negligence.

Civil law defences available in the law of torts

Contributory negligence is only a partial defence which reduces a claim for damages against a defendant by considering the plaintiff's role and contributing acts in the latter's injuries or damages.

Illegality can be raised as a defence when the defendant causes injury to the plaintiff while the latter is performing an illegal action. The general principle is that no one should benefit from a criminal enterprise.

Inevitable accident is a defence that will negate an offender's liability when the victim suffers injury as a result of an accident; ie an event that is beyond the defendant's control. An accident can be defined as a situation that cannot be avoided by any means or precautions that a reasonable person might be expected to take in the circumstances.

Mistake, ie a mistaken belief either of fact or law, is not a general defence and the significance of a mistake will vary from one case to another. A mistake that a reasonable man could have made in the same circumstances might be a defence.

Necessity is 'a mixture of charity, the maintenance of the public good and self-protection, and [the defence of necessity] is probably limited to cases involving an urgent situation of imminent peril'.[16] An action taken out of necessity must be justified by its reasonableness, which the court will assess on a case-by-case basis. The court will consider what has been done in the individual circumstances of the case, what might be deemed to be reasonable action in a given situation, in this day and age under such circumstances.

Self-defence An individual has a right to defend himself as long as the force used for that purpose is considered proportionate to the danger. What amounts to reasonable force is a question of fact which is assessed on an individual case-by-case basis.

Statutory authority Where a statute authorises an act, which without consent would normally amount to an offence of assault, battery, or false imprisonment, this act, if performed within the ambit of the Act's provisions, will not be an offence as the statute will provide a valid defence. For instance, the statutory power to detain the mentally ill provided by Section 3 Mental Health Act 1983 justifies the detention of people with a mental illness who represent a threat to themselves or to the public – without this provision, the detention would amount to the criminal offence and civil tort of false imprisonment and to unlawful deprivation of liberty contrary to Article 5 (right to liberty and security) Human Rights Act 1998.[17]

Volenti non fit injuria, also known as consent, implies that a person cannot cause injury to someone who is consenting to the risk. However, this idea is tempered by the fact that consent is not merely about knowing the risk, it is also about understanding it – if there is no real understanding of the risk then there can be no consent.

Consent (in relation to medical treatment)

'"Consent" is the voluntary and continuing permission of the patient to receive a particular treatment, based on an adequate knowledge of the purpose, nature, likely effects and risks of that treatment, including the likelihood of its success and any alternatives to it.'[18]

Consent is sought and should be given before any medical care, treatment or examination is performed on a patient. A person who administers medical treatment to a patient who has not given consent, or who has clearly refused to give their consent, could be liable under both civil and criminal law.

The rules for valid consent will vary according to the nature of the condition that needs treating, ie whether it is treatment for a physical or mental disorder (the latter being covered by the Mental Health Act 1983). However, in general, for consent to be valid, three elements are required:

a) *Generally, the person giving the consent must have the capacity*[19] *to do so.* Once it is established that the patient understands the particular situation, ie has capacity, their decision to consent or not is valid, whether the reasons behind the decision are (un)reasonable, (ir)rational, (un)known or (non)existent.

b) *Generally, the person must be sufficiently informed as to the nature, purpose, potential risks and consequences of the proposed treatments, as well as to any alternative therapeutic methods available.* For those to whom the Mental Health Act 1983 might apply, paragraph 14.13(a) Code of Practice provides that in relation to consent to treatment 'the patient must be informed, in terms which he is likely to understand, of the nature, purpose and likely effects of the treatment proposed'.

c) *Generally, the consent must be given freely and voluntarily.* For those to whom the Mental Health Act 1983 might apply, paragraph 15.12 Code of Practice provides that 'permission given under any unfair or undue pressure is not "consent"'. Moreover, patients must be advised of their right to withdraw their consent to a treatment at any time before it is undergone.

Under Section 8(1) Family Law Reform Act 1969, the consent to surgical, medical and dental treatment of a child of 16 years of age is presumed to be an effective consent at law and no parental consent is necessary. Since *Gillick v West Norfolk and Wisbech AHA* in 1986,[20] it is recognised that a child under 16 can be legally capable of giving consent to a treatment if they show enough maturity, intelligence and comprehension as to the nature and implications of such a treatment.

Although it is acknowledged that parents are often the best judges as to what is in the best interest of their child, in some rare cases, the doctor might be the one best qualified to make that judgement. Where the parents refuse the treatment felt by the doctor to be in the child's best interests and the child is not deemed capable of providing the relevant consent, then the doctor must seek a court order known as a 'specific issue' order under Section 8 Children Act 1989 to sanction proceeding with the treatment in the absence of such consent. The court in such circumstances will hear all the evidence and will decide the case on the basis of what is in the child's paramount interests (Section 1(1) Children Act 1989).

Criminal law

A developed, civilised society will generally provide that certain types of conduct will not be acceptable and will provide for that conduct to be unlawful through its criminal law. The criminal law of England and Wales is made up of offences to be found either in statutes passed by Parliament or in judge-made or customary law referred to as the 'common law'.

In broad terms, the criminal law of England and Wales requires that before a person can be convicted it must be proved *beyond reasonable doubt* that the person has acted in a way which is deemed criminal (the deed of *actus reus*) *and that the person has acted intentionally* or *recklessly* as to the consequences (the mental element or the *mens rea*). There are criminal offences, offences of *strict liability*, which do not require proof of a mental element, but these do not relate to any of the actions described in this guide.

In contrast with civil law where a private individual may take the initiative to present an action before the courts, in criminal law the Police will consider charging the alleged offender and the Crown Prosecution Service – the government department responsible for prosecuting an offence through the courts – on behalf of the State, will consider bringing a prosecution against any individual who has committed an unlawful criminal act. If found guilty in the courts after trial or after a plea of guilty, the offender will then be sentenced. The sentence can be one of imprisonment, a fine, a compensation order, or a community rehabilitation or punishment order.

Where any person therefore engages in any sort of conduct which has been designated a 'criminal offence', and the Police are notified, they will then investigate and consider charging the individual concerned with the particular criminal offence. If the Police encounter some difficulties in, for instance, the investigation of a suspected false imprisonment, or assault and/or battery against a child, young person or adult with a learning disability and presenting severe challenging behaviour, they may want to refer the case to the Crown Prosecution Service for advice. The Crown Prosecution Service will then consider all the circumstances of the case and will pay special attention to whether the facts disclosed that give rise to possible charges by the Police are actually justified by such defences as self-defence, action taken to prevent the commission of a crime etc.

Criminal law offences include: false imprisonment, common assault, battery, assault occasioning bodily harm, Section 18 Offences Against the Person Act 1861 malicious wounding/inflicting grievous bodily harm with intent to cause grievous bodily harm, Section 20 Offences Against the Person Act 1861 wounding/causing grievous bodily harm without intent to cause grievous bodily harm, murder, voluntary manslaughter and involuntary manslaughter.

Criminal law defences

1) Common law and statutory power to detain the insane   There is no power at common law to apprehend or detain a person suffering from mental disorder simply because he is so suffering. But it is stated that a 'private person may without express warrant confine a person disordered in his mind who seems disposed to do mischief to himself or any other person'.[21] While it is accepted that this power derives from a rather old judicial authority (going back more than 100 years) it is submitted that it would be untenable for the criminal law to provide no protection for an individual with severe learning disabilities presenting severe challenging behaviour.

Statutory power – Section 3(1) and (2) of the Mental Health Act 1983 stipulates that a patient may be admitted to a hospital and detained there for the period allowed by the provisions of this Act if the patient is suffering from a mental illness or another mental disorder which demands medical treatment in a hospital; and if it is necessary for the patient's health and safety, as well as for the safety of others that he is detained under this Act.

2) Consent As a general principle, when the victim has given consent then there is no offence. In cases where consent is given to an unlawful use of force, which does not result in causing injury, the defence will be upheld. However, in *Donovan* 1934,[22] it was held that an assault 'cannot be rendered lawful because the person to whose detriment it is done consents to it. No person can license another to commit a crime'.

3) Duress of circumstances, which is not available as defence for murder or attempted murder, may be raised as a defence where a person argues that they may have had to perform an act under the pressure of certain circumstances. This will be valid as a defence if it can be proven that the defendant acted in a reasonable manner, applying only the necessary amount of force to avoid a threat of injury or death.

4) Lawful correction is a defence available, but note since implementation of Section 58 Children Act 2004 on 15 January 2005 the law is different in that it restricts the defence of reasonable punishment only to a charge of common assault. Before implementation of the Children Act 2004 Section 58, the defence was theoretically available to any offence charged where the parent claimed lawful correction available to parents in England and Wales who have the right to dispense corporal punishment to their child, for whom they have parental responsibility. The defence will be valid provided the punishment is 'reasonable'. The standards of reasonableness have changed over the years. Thus judges have adopted a different approach to the question of reasonableness according to the standards current at the time of trial. When directing a jury, at present, as influenced by the decisions of the European Court of Human Rights, a 'reasonable' punishment will imply that a) it is not immoderate and excessive; b) it is not for the satisfaction of a parent's personal gratification; c) it is not beyond the child's endurance; c) it is not administered by an inappropriate instrument likely to threaten the child's life and integrity of limbs; and d) the child understands the nature of the punishment.

In accordance with the judgement of the European Court of Human Rights,[23] in *R v H (Assault of Child: Reasonable Chastisement)* 2002[24] it was held that when assessing the reasonableness of a chastisement, a judge, in giving directions to the jury or in determining sentence in the case of a plea of guilty, should consider: the nature and context of the behaviour of the person being chastised; the duration of the punishment; its physical and mental consequences in relation to the child; the age and personal characteristics of the child; and the reasons given by the adult for administering punishment.

Pursuant to Section 131 Schools Standards and Framework Act 1998, no member of any staff in any educational institution has the right to administer corporal punishment to pupils under any circumstances. Parents cannot delegate this responsibility to any such person employed in a school even where they argue it is in accordance with their religious beliefs (see also *Williamson v Secretary of State for Education and Employment* 2003[25]).

5) Mistake In order for mistake to succeed as a defence, it must be based on the facts of the circumstances as the defendant saw them or believed them to be. If the mistake is genuine, albeit unreasonable, the defendant will be allowed to raise it as a defence.

6) Necessity could be described as a situation where a person has to make a choice between two courses of action, both of which would result in some kind of harm being caused. However, the choice of which course of action is best must take into consideration which of these would cause the lesser harm. Necessity can be a defence in cases: a) where a person has no choice but to act in such a way in order to protect themselves; b) when the defendant performs an 'illegal' act to save someone's life; and c) involving issues of mental capacity and consent, where a decision to save or assist someone's life without their consent has to be made.

7) Prevention of a breach of the peace In a caring situation, a carer could use this defence where a person with learning disabilities whom she cares for is restrained because they are likely to cause harm to other individuals or property in the immediate future, or where harm is feared in the immediate future *as a result of* an affray, a riot, assault or other disturbance. It would not make a restraint lawful where it is used to prevent the person with learning disabilities harming themselves.

A situation where there is public alarm or general excitement will not constitute a breach of the peace unless there is an actual or potential threat of violence that is likely to occur in the near future.

8) Prevention of crime Section 3(1) Criminal Law Act 1967 stipulates that 'a person may use such force as is reasonable in the circumstances in the prevention of a crime. . .'. A crime, in this context, could be an unlawful act that is about or likely to incur physical damage to an individual or to property. This defence, which is really only a justification for the commission of an unlawful act, can only be used for offences where some degree of force is employed.

9) Self-defence This defence encompasses actions taken to defend oneself as well as another from being the victim of an unlawful attack on their person (Section 3 Criminal Act 1967), although it will not be available if the force is used after all danger has disappeared.

The use of force must be reasonable as regards the danger; so if it is disproportionate, ie excessive, then the defence will not be available. Paradoxically, the belief in having to use force in self-defence need not be reasonable, as the facts of the circumstances must be assessed in the light of what the defendant believed them to be. In other words, the court will consider the fact that the defendant acted honestly and instinctively doing what he thought was necessary in the circumstances as strong evidence to support the defence. If, based upon the facts as seen by the defendant, a reasonable person would have acted in the same way, then the defence is likely to succeed. If a reasonable person would not have acted in the same way, then the defence will fail.

Disability

Section 1(1) Disability Discrimination Act 1995 provides that 'a person has a disability for the purposes of this Act if he has a physical or mental impairment which has a substantial and long-term adverse effect on his ability to carry out normal day-to-day activities'. A disabled person, therefore, means someone who has a disability.

Employer's responsibility

In tort law, an employer can be found liable for the act of his employees even though he is not the tortfeasor, ie the person actually committing the wrong. Vicarious liability involves imposing liability on the employer for the act of his employees, done in the course of their employment. Employer's liability is concerned with rendering the employer accountable for any breach of his duty of care towards his employees.

Human Rights Act 1998

The Human Rights Act 1998 (implemented 2 October 2000), provides a structure for the protection of individuals' rights before the national courts, and a procedure through which they can claim a remedy against the State or one of its representatives (public bodies) for breaches of provisions of the European Convention on Human Rights. Actions under the Act can only be brought against a public authority, not against a private individual. However, the national courts are nonetheless under an obligation to interpret the law in accordance with the Convention, which means that Convention rights can be invoked (and thus must be respected) in an action involving private parties.

Lawful excuse

There will be many situations in which parents or carers of children and young people, or the parents or the adult children of adults with learning disabilities who also present severe challenging behaviour, technically commit criminal and/or civil offences. This may come about in an attempt to provide adequate care, control and safety of their children, be they under 18 or adults, or for their parents, or to provide for the safety of other persons.

The notion of 'lawful excuse' is referred to in cases where a carer's conduct is justified in the eyes of the law. Without this lawful excuse, the carer's conduct would normally constitute a criminal offence or civil wrong. A lawful excuse thus acts as a defence to a potential criminal or civil liability.

There is, however, no statutory and clear definition of what constitutes a lawful excuse. The general essence remains that a lawful excuse justifies a conduct, which would otherwise be unlawful and would give rise to a liability. However, a lawful excuse will vary according to situations to which it applies.

For instance, in a recent UK Parliament session, members of the Lords discussed the issue of defining 'lawful excuse/authority' with regards to an Animal Health Bill.[26] Lord Plumb argued that it 'should . . . be defined in the legislation in order for anyone to go to court and use it as a defence'. Lord Whitty stated:

> '*Lawful authority* is normally powers given by statute; a *lawful excuse* is one which could be legally proven in court as a reason for not complying with an order. If we go back to *reasonableness, mitigating circumstances* and so on, that is what *excuse* means. But *authority* would be something that is statutorily based...'.

Section 5(2) Criminal Damage Act 1971 provides that a person who damages another's property would have a lawful excuse if at the time of the damage he believed that the owner of the damaged property actually consented to the destruction of his property or would have done so given the circumstances, or that the offender acted in that way in order to protect another's property, ie his own or somebody else's, and that such action was reasonable.

For details on the various lawful excuses, see the section on the civil and criminal law defences.

Learning difficulty

Section 312 Part IV Education Act 1996 provides that:

> '*a child has a learning difficulty if:*
>
> (a) *he has a significantly greater difficulty in learning than the majority of children of his age,*
>
> (b) *he has a disability which either prevents or hinders him from making use of educational facilities of a kind generally provided for children of his age in schools within the area of the local education authority, or*
>
> (c) *he is under the age of five and is, or would be if special educational provision were not made for him, likely to fall within paragraph (a) or (b) when of or over that age.*'

Learning disability

There is no statutory definition of learning disability; however, this expression is seen by some as equating with the term 'mental impairment', defined further below.

Medical treatment

Certain 'psychoactive' and 'anti-psychotic' medications are used in the treatment of challenging behaviours. There are various forms of psychotropic drugs, such as antipsychotics, anxiolytics, anti-manics, anti-depressants, anti-epileptics, stimulants and opiate antagonists, which were originally used in cases of mental illness such as schizophrenia.[27]

These drugs have been progressively and widely used to manage challenging situations despite some studies showing that they are not very effective in this domain as it is argued that there is a lack of relationship between challenging behaviour and mental illness. Nevertheless, psychotropic drugs are still used, either as part of a therapeutic treatment or in an emergency situation. In the case of a therapeutic treatment, the issue of consent is raised, and with it, the question of capacity. In the case of an emergency use of the medication, the possible offence of battery becomes an issue.

Mental impairment

Section 1 of the Mental Health Act 1983 provides a definition of 'mental impairment', which is a 'state of arrested or incomplete development of mind which includes significant impairment of intelligence and social functioning'.

Parent

The parents of a child are either the biological parents, ie the child was produced from the female's egg and male's sperm and carried by the female, or they are people who are treated as the mother and father as defined by the Human Fertilisation and Embryology Act 1990.

Section 27(1) defines a mother as: 'the woman who is carrying or has carried a child as a result of the placing in her of an embryo or of sperm and eggs and no other woman is to be treated as mother of the child'.

Section 28(2) states that a father is 'a man who is married to the mother and did not object to the placing in her of the embryo or the sperm and eggs or to her insemination', and

Section 28(3) makes the same provision as above but for an unmarried couple. No other man is to be treated as the father of the child.

Parental responsibility

The Children Act 1989 provides specifically that parents have *responsibilities*, not rights. However, Section 3(1) Children Act 1989 defines parental responsibility as: 'All the rights, duties, powers, responsibilities and authority which by law a parent of a child has in relation to the child and his property'. The Act does not actually define these rights, duties, powers and responsibilities. The Department of Health's Introduction to the Children Act 1989 points out that: 'that choice of words emphasises that: "the duty to care for the child and to raise him to moral, physical and emotional health and it is the fundamental task of parenthood and the only justification for the authority that it confers".'

Who holds parental responsibility?

- *Married parents:* both mother and father

- *Unmarried parents:* mother alone unless father has taken formal legal steps to acquire, and has acquired parental responsibility

- *Divorced:* both even if child lives with one parent

- *Persons holding a Section 8 Children Act 1989 residence order:* but in the case of non-parents only for the duration of the order (Section 12(2) Children Act 1989)

Who does not hold parental responsibility?

- *Unmarried fathers:* unless he registered the child's birth, applies for a court order or makes a formal agreement with the mother on a special form lodged with the appropriate court offices. Since the implementation on December 1, 2003, of the amendment made to Section 4 of the Children Act 1989 by the Adoption and Children Act 2002, unmarried fathers have been able for the first time to acquire parental responsibility where they register the child's birth together with the mother. This amendment, however, only applies to those fathers registering the child's birth after 1 December 2003. Thus, those unmarried fathers who had registered the child's birth before that date will still have to make an agreement with the mother or apply to the court for an order under Section 4 Children Act 1989.

- *Step-parents:* unless conferred through Section 8 residence order under the Children Act or adoption (NB After implementation of the relevant provisions of the Adoption and Children Act 2002 (as yet no date has been set) step-parents will be able to apply for parental responsibility orders under the newly inserted Section 4A Children Act 1989.

Parental responsibility (revoking of)

Parental responsibility can be revoked on the a) death of the child; b) upon adoption; c) freeing for adoption; d) the court revoking a parental responsibility order under Section 4 Children Act 1989; and e) on the discharge of a residence order held by someone other than a parent.

Exercise of parental responsibility

Parental responsibility including, for example the responsibility to give consent for medical operations or the administration of medication, *can* be exercised by one parent possessed of parental responsibility unless it is consent for: a) adoption; b) marriage; and/or c) freeing for adoption, in which case both parents, where they both have parental responsibility, will have to give consent or their consent will have to be dispensed with. Parents, or those with parental responsibility, *cannot* act in a way which is contrary to an order made under the 1989 Children Act, ie if an order has been made that a child must go to a special therapy unit, the father cannot stop the child going.

Parents *can delegate responsibility* to, for example, childminders, carers and/or schools.

Parents may be found to be negligent if, knowing their child to be prone to severe challenging behaviour, they place the care of their child in the hands of a person lacking sufficient skill, experience or qualifications to look after such a child. If any injury befell the child of a third party (ie another child) caused by the inexperience of the carer, parents may bear responsibility and thus may be sued for damages.

In practice, most parents would not be insured against such risks and therefore it would not be considered worthwhile bringing an action against them, more particularly if the action were being considered on behalf of their own child. However, the parents of another child to whom injury has been caused may feel that it is worth their while pursuing legal action in anticipation of recovering even a small award for damages to compensate their child for any injuries received and any consequential additional costs.

Once a child attains the age of 18, then the parent no longer has parental responsibility even where the adult child lacks decision-making capacity. (Note – changes will occur in this situation once the Mental Capacity Bill, currently before Parliament, is enacted.)

Physical intervention

As is pointed out in the *Guidance on the Use of Physical Interventions* (DoH/DfES 2002) there are different forms of physical intervention, which are summarised in the table below (taken from paragraph 3.1 of that Guidance).

	Bodily contact	Mechanical	Environmental change
Non-restrictive	Manual guidance to assist a person walking	Use of a protective helmet to prevent self injury	Removal of the cause of distress, for example, adjusting temperature, light or background noise
Restrictive	Holding a person's hands to prevent them from hitting someone	Use of arm cuffs or splints to prevent self injury	Forcible seclusion or the use of locked doors

The Guidance states that the:

> 'table shows the difference between restrictive forms of physical intervention which are designed to prevent movement or mobility or to disengage from dangerous or harmful physical contact, and non-restrictive methods. Restrictive physical interventions involve the use of force to control a person's behaviour and can be employed using bodily contact, mechanical devices or changes to the person's environment. The use of force is associated with increased risks regarding the safety of service users and staff and inevitably affects personal freedom and choice.' (paragraph 3.1)

Positive handling

This is a term used by some to describe a whole plan which has been devised for the child, young person or adult which may incorporate physical intervention strategies and which may also include other systems of rewards as reinforcement of good behaviour. It is also used by others simply as an alternative term to the expression 'physical intervention' because it does not have the same negative connotations as the latter term and therefore may be more acceptable both to those dealing with children and adults with learning disabilities and severe challenging behaviour and to their parents.

Although 'positive handling' is mentioned in paragraph 8.2 of the DoH/DfES *Guidance on the Use of Physical Interventions* – in which it is stated that 'in schools, the possible use of restrictive physical interventions, as part of a broader educational or therapeutic strategy, will be included within the pupil's *Positive Handling Plan*' – there is no definition of this term anywhere in this Guidance.

Restrictive physical intervention (RPI)

Restrictive physical intervention, as set out in paragraph 3.1 of the *Guidance on the Use of Physical Interventions*, is defined as involving 'the use of force to control a person's behaviour and can be employed using bodily contact, mechanical devices, or changes to the person's environment'.

Risk assessment

Under Health and Safety legislation employers are required to conduct suitable and sufficient assessment of risks to the health and safety of employees when they are at work, and of people who are not in employment but who might be affected by the employers/employees' actions or work activity. According to paragraph 1.5 of the *Guidance on the Use of Physical Interventions*, risk assessment should be carried out in the same way in relation to people who present challenging behaviours. Thus there must be an assessment of the risks which the behaviour of such people may present to employees, as well as to people who are not in employment and who might be affected by the person's behaviour. For example, this might include the risks to other people and any visitors.

Social care worker

Section 55(2) Care Standards Act 2000 provides that a 'social care worker' is a person who:

'*(a) engages in relevant social work (referred to in this Part as a 'social worker');*

(b) is employed at a children's home, care home or residential family centre or for the purposes of a domiciliary care agency, a fostering agency or a voluntary adoption agency;

(c) manages an establishment, or an agency, of a description mentioned in paragraph (b) or,

(d) is supplied by a domiciliary care agency to provide personal care in their own homes for persons who by reason of illness, infirmity or disability are unable to provide it for themselves without assistance.'

Section 55(3) also stipulates that the following people are to be treated as 'social care workers':

'(a) a person engaged in work for the purposes of a local authority's social services functions, or in the provision of services similar to services which may or must be provided by local authorities in the exercise of those functions;

(b) a person engaged in the provision of personal care for any person;

(c) a person who manages, or is employed in, an undertaking (other than an establishment or agency) which consists of or includes supplying, or providing services for the purpose of supplying, persons to provide personal care;

(d) a person employed in connection with the discharge of functions of the appropriate Minister under section 80 of the 1989 Act (inspection of children's homes etc);

(e) staff of the Commission or the Assembly who:

(i) inspect premises under section 87 of the 1989 Act (welfare of children accommodated in independent schools and colleges) or section 31 or 45 of this Act; or

(ii) are responsible for persons who do so;

and staff of the Assembly who inspect premises under section 79 of that Act (inspection of child minding and day care in Wales) or are responsible for persons who do so;

(f) a person employed in a day centre;

(g) a person participating in a course approved by a Council under section 63 for persons wishing to become social workers.'

Finally, Section 55(4) defines 'relevant social work' as 'social work which is required in connection with any health, education or social services provided by any person'; and Section 55(5) describes a 'day centre' as a place where nursing or personal care (but not accommodation) is provided wholly or mainly for persons mentioned in Section 3(2).

Supply worker

Section 80(5) Care Standards Act 2000 defines a supply worker as someone who:

> *'(a) in relation to an employment agency, means an individual supplied by the agency for employment in a care position or for whom the agency has found employment in a care position;*
>
> *(b) in relation to an employment business, means an individual supplied by the business for employment in a care position.'*

Vulnerable adult

Section 80(6) Care Standards Act 2000 defines a vulnerable adult as:

> *'(a) an adult to whom accommodation and nursing or personal care are provided in a care home;*
>
> *(b) an adult to whom personal care is provided in their own home under arrangements made by a domiciliary care agency; or*
>
> *(c) an adult to whom prescribed services are provided by an independent hospital, independent clinic, independent medical agency or National Health Service body.'*

There is, as yet, no comparable definition of a vulnerable child.

References

[1] *Guidance on the Use of Physical Interventions*, Department for Education and Employment, SEN (Special Educational Needs), July 2002, http://www.dfes.gov.uk/sen/documents/PI_Guidance.pdf

[2] *Five Steps to Risk Assessment*, HSE Books, weblink: http://www.hse.gov.uk/pubns/indg163.pdf

[3] For a step-by-step risk assessment tailored to situations involving the management of challenging behaviours, refer to David Allen's *Ethical Approaches to Physical Interventions – Responding to Challenging Behaviour in People with Intellectual Disabilities*, BILD 2003

[4] http://www.doh.gov.uk/violencetaskforce/card.htm

[5] (2002) 35 European Human Rights Reports 1 European Court of Human Rights

[6] (1999) 27 European Human Rights Reports 611

[7] *Positive Behavioural Management – Preventing & Responding to Aggressive Behaviour in Persons with Intellectual Disabilities*, Trainer's Manual, PRT, 1999, unit 10 – Crisis, Self Protected Strategies, (10.30 section 6)

[8] This means sit in a room and observe the person, answering to his needs (eg drinks, food)

[9] Section 2, paragraph 2.5, at p.9 – DoH 2003 http://www.doh.gov.uk/pdfs/nosecrets.pdf

[10] Caring About Carers, http://www.carers.gov.uk/whatis.htm

[11] Caring About Carers, http://www.carers.gov.uk/whatis.htm, April 2003, DoH. According to this website, there are approximately 5.7 million people who fit this definition in the UK today. In *Caring about Carers* the Government made a commitment to provide details of the services or benefits affecting carers on the Internet

[12] *Valuing People*, chapter 2, pp.23–26, DoH 2001

[13] Emerson E, *Challenging Behaviour Analysis and Intervention in People with Learning Disabilities*. Cambridge: Cambridge University Press 1995

[14] The Mental Health Foundation, *Don't Forget Us – Children with Learning Disabilities and Severe Challenging Behaviour*, 1997, p.12

[15] Martin E A (ed), *Oxford Dictionary of Law*, Oxford University Press, 2002

[16] Rogers W V H, *Winfield & Jolowicz on Tort*, 16th edition, London & Maxwell 2002, p.872

[17] See appendix at p.31 for full details of the article

[18] Department of Health and Welsh Office, *Code of Practice, Mental Health Act 1983*, published August 1993, paragraph 15.12

[19] See definition of capacity, p.36

[20] [1986] AC 112

[21] Bacon's Abridgement cited in Hoggett B, *Mental Health Law* (Sweet & Maxwell, 2000)

[22] [1934] 2 KB 498

[23] *A v United Kingdom* (1999) 27 European Human Rights Reports 611

[24] [2002] 1 Cr.App.R.7

[25] [2003] 1 F.L.R. 726. (Note this case has gone on appeal to the House of Lords) This decision covers children, of whatever age, in any form of private or state-funded education

[26] 8 Oct 2002: Column 225, http://www.parliament.the-stationery-office.co.uk/pa/ld199900/ldhansrd/pdvn/lds02/text/21008-23.htm

[27] Kennedy C H and Meyer K A, The Use of Psychotropic Medication for People with Severe Disabilities and Challenging Behaviour: current status and future directions, *Journal of the Association for Persons with Severe Handicaps*, 23, 1998, pp.83–97